Dietary Supplements and Multiple Sclerosis: A Health Professional's Guide

Allen C. Bowling, MD, PhD

Medical Director and Director of
Complementary and Alternative Medicine,
Rocky Mountain Multiple Sclerosis Center, Englewood, Colorado

Clinical Associate Professor of Neurology,
University of Colorado Health Sciences Center, Denver, Colorado

Thomas M. Stewart, JD, PA-C

Associate Director of Complementary
and Alternative Medicine,
Rocky Mountain Multiple Sclerosis Center, Englewood, Colorado

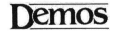

New York

Contents

Appendices

Acknowledgments

It was possible to write this book through the support of several individuals and organizations. The Rocky Mountain Multiple Sclerosis Center has provided ongoing support for the Complementary and Alternative Medicine Program that is based at the Center. For this particular project, Serono, Inc. provided valuable support, Drew S. Kern assisted with the word processing, and Dr. Diana M. Schneider at Demos Medical Publishing provided helpful suggestions. Finally, we thank our families for tolerating the time that we spent researching and writing the manuscript.

Serono, Inc. provided an educational grant to support this publication but Serono, Inc. and Pfizer Inc. do not endorse any specific treatment discussed in this book.

Introduction

This book is for health professionals who care for people with multiple sclerosis (MS). There is a relatively high use of complementary and alternative medicine (CAM), especially dietary supplements, among people with MS. Conventional health professionals are in a potentially valuable position to be a trustworthy source of objective information about CAM to their patients. However, many patients do not discuss their use of CAM during their conventional medical appointments, and many health professionals do not have the knowledge base to discuss these therapies. This book is designed to fill the knowledge gap in the area of MS-relevant dietary supplements and thereby foster communication about CAM between people with MS and health professionals.

This book is meant to be kept in the clinic and referred to when people with MS ask a question about a particular dietary supplement. The supplements are arranged in alphabetical order under the most commonly used name. In addition, the index contains a listing of these common names as well as less common names that may be encountered. The main information about the supplements is written in a concise summary form that usually discusses only the MS relevance of the supplement. References and additional reading sources are also provided for each supplement that is reviewed. For supplements that are more likely to be used because of possible efficacy or popularity, additional information is provided about dosages, interactions with drugs and other dietary supplements, contraindications (relative and absolute), and side effects (even more detailed information can be found in the references and additional reading provided at the end of each listing). With the information arranged in this manner, health professionals should be able to provide information about several supplements quickly during the course of a routine office visit.

The supplements that are reviewed in this guide were chosen by several criteria. Supplements are included that have specific MS relevance (such as those that are known to be used by people with MS) have claimed

efficacy for slowing disease progression or relieving MS symptoms, interact with drugs commonly used to treat MS, and potentially worsen MS or
its symptoms. Also, supplements are reviewed that are popular in the general population or are known to have serious adverse effects.

There are many potential benefits for health professionals who develop
a knowledge base, interest in, and openness to CAM. The area of CAM may
be fascinating and may encourage health professionals to think about treatment from the patient's perspective and to consider alternative ways of
understanding MS pathogenesis and treatment. Health professionals with
CAM information can improve the quality of patient care by guiding patients
away from possibly harmful therapies and, if appropriate, toward low-risk,
possibly effective therapies. It is hoped that patients will appreciate being
able to discuss CAM therapies openly with health professionals and will
regard health professionals as sources of unbiased CAM information.

Using this guide in the course of a medical visit can be a time-effi-
cient way to build a base of CAM knowledge. As noted, the information in
this guide is meant to be concise and MS-relevant. To complement this
information, broader based information about dietary supplements and
other forms of CAM can be found in a variety of sources, some of which
are listed below. These references, which we have cited frequently, were
extremely helpful in writing this book.

Dietary supplements generally
Fetrow CW, Avila JR. *Professional's Handbook of Complementary & Alternative
    Medicines*. 2nd ed. Springhouse, PA: Springhouse Corp, 2001.
Fragakis AS. *The Health Professional's Guide to Popular Dietary Supplements*. 2nd ed.
    Chicago, IL: American Dietetic Association, 2003.
Jellin JM, Gregory PJ, Batz F, et al. *Pharmacist's Letter/Prescriber's Letter Natural
    Medicines Comprehensive Database*. 4th ed. Stockton, CA: Therapeutic
    Research Faculty, 2002.

CAM and MS
Bowling AC. *Alternative Medicine and Multiple Sclerosis*. New York: Demos Medical
    Publishing, Inc., 2001.
Bowling AC, Ibrahim R, Stewart TM. Alternative medicine and multiple sclerosis: an
    objective review from an American perspective. *Int J MS Care* 2000; 2:14–21.
Bowling AC, Stewart TM. Current complementary and alternative therapies for
    multiple sclerosis. *Curr Treat Options Neurol* 2003; 5:55–68.
www.ms-cam.org: CAM website of the Rocky Mountain MS Center; contains
    detailed, referenced, evidence-based reviews of MS-relevant CAM.

CAM generally
Ernst E, Pittler MH, Stevinson C, White A. *The Desktop Guide to Complementary
    and Alternative Medicine: An Evidence-Based Approach*. London: Harcourt
    Publishers Limited, 2001.

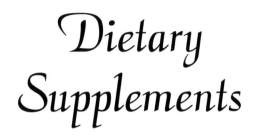

Dietary Supplements

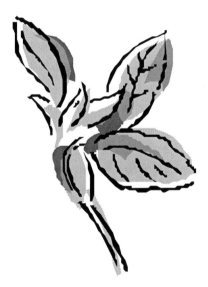

Dietary Supplements

5-HTP

Other names: 5-hydroxytryptophan

SUMMARY: Although 5-HTP is possibly effective for treating depression, it should be avoided since, like L-tryptophan, it may cause eosinophilia-myalgia syndrome.

References and additional reading:

Jellin JM, Gregory PJ, Batz F, et al. *Pharmacist's Letter/Prescriber's Letter Natural Medicines Comprehensive Database.* 4th ed. Stockton, CA: Therapeutic Research Faculty, 2002:11–12.

ALFALFA

Other names: buffalo herb, lucerne, phytoestrogen

SUMMARY: Due to the possible immune-stimulating effects of L-canavanine, a component of alfalfa, this herb poses a theoretical risk in MS and may decrease the effectiveness of immune-modulating and immune-suppressing therapies.

References and additional reading:

Brinker F. *Herb Contraindications and Drug Interactions.* Sandy, OR: Eclectic Medical Publications, 1998:27–28.

Fetrow CW, Avila JR. *Professional's Handbook of Complementary & Alternative Medicines.* 2nd ed. Springhouse, PA: Springhouse Corp, 2001:24–26.

Jellin JM, Gregory PJ, Batz F, et al. *Pharmacist's Letter/Prescriber's Letter Natural Medicines Comprehensive Database.* 4th ed. Stockton, CA: Therapeutic Research Faculty, 2002:35–36.

Newall CA, Anderson LA, Phillipson JD. *Herbal Medicines: A Guide for Health-Care Professionals*. London: The Pharmaceutical Press, 1996:23–24.

Peirce A. *Practical Guide to Natural Medicines*. New York: The Stonesong Press, 1999:26–27.

ALOE (oral use)

Other names: aloe vera, burn plant, lily of the desert, miracle plant, plant of immortality

SUMMARY: Due to the presence of anthracene derivatives, aloe has laxative effects. It is sometimes recommended for MS, but there are no studies documenting its efficacy for MS. It may potentiate the hypokalemic effects of steroids. Also, oral use in general is not recommended due to multiple possible adverse effects, including abdominal pain, diarrhea, damage to the intestinal mucosa, nephritis, hypokalemia, hematuria, muscle weakness, cardiac arrhythmias, spontaneous abortion, and premature birth.

References and additional reading:

Brinker F. *Herb Contraindications and Drug Interactions*. Sandy, OR: Eclectic Medical Publications, 1998:28–30.

Duke JA, Bogenschutz-Godwin MJ, duCellier J, Duke P-AK. *Handbook of Medicinal Herbs*. 2nd ed. Boca Raton, FL: CRC Press, 2002:17–18.

Ernst E, Pittler MH, Stevinson C, White A. *The Desktop Guide to Complementary and Alternative Medicine: An Evidence-Based Approach*. London: Harcourt Publishers Limited, 2001:84–85.

Fetrow CW, Avila JR. *Professional's Handbook of Complementary & Alternative Medicines*. 2nd ed. Springhouse, PA: Springhouse Corp, 2001:29–32.

Jellin JM, Gregory PJ, Batz F, et al. *Pharmacist's Letter/Prescriber's Letter Natural Medicines Comprehensive Database*. 4th ed. Stockton, CA: Therapeutic Research Faculty, 2002:39–41.

Newall CA, Anderson LA, Phillipson JD. *Herbal Medicines: A Guide for Health-Care Professionals*. London: The Pharmaceutical Press, 1996:25–26.

Peirce A. *Practical Guide to Natural Medicines*. New York: The Stonesong Press, 1999:31–35.

Schulz V, Hänsel R, Tyler VE. *Rational Phytotherapy: A Physicians' Guide to Herbal Medicine*. 3rd ed. Berlin: Springer-Verlag, 1998:210–211.

ALPHA-LIPOIC ACID

Other names: ALA, lipoic acid, thioctic acid

SUMMARY: One study reports that alpha-lipoic acid (ALA) decreases T-cell migration into the spinal cord and inhibits matrix metalloproteinase-9, an enzyme involved in T-cell trafficking. ALA reduces disease severity in experimental allergic encephalomyelitis (EAE). These studies are encouraging, but human clinical studies are needed to determine if ALA is an effective treatment for MS. ALA has diverse effects on the immune system; some studies indicate immune-stimulating effects that could pose theoretical risks in MS and antagonize the effects of immune-suppressing and immune-modulating drugs.

Additional information:

Dosage: of note, I.V. use may be required for therapeutic effects; 20–50 mg P.O. daily as a general antioxidant; 800–1800 mg P.O. daily or 100–1200 mg I.V. daily have been used in clinical trials of peripheral and autonomic neuropathies

Contraindications and warnings: diabetes (hypoglycemic effect), bleeding disorders (intravenous use), pregnancy and lactation (insufficient information)

Major interactions: oral hypoglycemic medications, insulin

Main side effects: skin rash, nausea, vomiting, headache, bleeding disorders (intravenous use)

References and additional reading:

Bowling AC. *Alternative Medicine and Multiple Sclerosis.* New York: Demos Medical Publishing, Inc., 2001:198–199.

Bowling AC, Stewart TM. Current complementary and alternative therapies for multiple sclerosis. *Curr Treat Options Neurol* 2003;5:55–68.

Fragakis AS. *The Health Professional's Guide to Popular Dietary Supplements.* 2nd ed. Chicago, IL: American Dietetic Association, 2003:11–16.

Jellin JM, Gregory PJ, Batz F, et al. *Pharmacist's Letter/Prescriber's Letter Natural Medicines Comprehensive Database.* 4th ed. Stockton, CA: Therapeutic Research Faculty, 2002:47–49.

Marcucci GH, Jones RE, McKeon GP, et al. Alpha lipoic acid inhibits T cell migration into the spinal cord and suppresses and treats experimental autoimmune encephalomyelitis. *J Neuroimmunol* 2002;131:104–114.

Ohmori H, Yamauchi T, Yamamoto I. Augmentation of the antibody response by lipoic acid in mice. II. Restoration of the antibody response in immunosuppressed mice. *Jap J Pharmacol* 1986;42:275–280.

Pack RA, Hardy K, Madigan MC, et al. Differential effects of the antioxidant alphalipoic acid on the proliferation of mitogen-stimulated peripheral blood lymphocytes and leukaemic T cells. *Mol Immunol* 2002;38:733–745.

ANDROSTENEDIONE

Other names: 4–androstene-3,17–dione, andro, androstene

SUMMARY: Androstenedione is sometimes claimed to improve energy, strength, and sexual function, but there is no evidence of efficacy and it may cause serious side effects. In women, it may cause masculinization, depression, and increased risk of breast cancer. In men, possible side effects include decreased spermatogenesis; testicular atrophy; gynecomastia; behavioral changes; and increased risk of prostate cancer, pancreatic cancer, and heart disease.

References and additional reading:

Fetrow CW, Avila JR. *Professional's Handbook of Complementary & Alternative Medicines.* 2nd ed. Springhouse, PA: Springhouse Corp, 2001:34–37.

Fragakis AS. *The Health Professional's Guide to Popular Dietary Supplements.* 2nd ed. Chicago, IL: American Dietetic Association, 2003:16–20.

Jellin JM, Gregory PJ, Batz F, et al. *Pharmacist's Letter/Prescriber's Letter Natural Medicines Comprehensive Database.* 4th ed. Stockton, CA: Therapeutic Research Faculty, 2002:72–73.

ASCORBIC ACID: see vitamin C

ASHWAGANDHA

Other names: Ayurvedic ginseng, Indian ginseng, winter cherry, withania

SUMMARY: This ayurvedic herb is sometimes recommended for MS. However, it has immune-stimulating effects that pose theoretical risks in MS and may interfere with the effectiveness of immune-modulating and immunosuppressive medications. Also, it has sedating properties that may worsen MS fatigue or potentiate the sedating effects of medications.

References and additional reading:

Jellin JM, Gregory PJ, Batz F, et al. *Pharmacist's Letter/Prescriber's Letter Natural Medicines Comprehensive Database.* 4th ed. Stockton, CA: Therapeutic Research Faculty, 2002:98–100.

Peirce A. *Practical Guide to Natural Medicines.* New York: The Stonesong Press, 1999:49–51.

ASIAN GINSENG

Other names: Chinese ginseng, ginseng root, Japanese ginseng, panax ginseng

SUMMARY: There is limited evidence that this herb may mildly improve cognitive function and prevent the common cold and flu. However, its use has never been studied in MS cognitive dysfunction, it may interact with steroids and stimulant medications, and its immune-stimulating effects pose theoretical risks in MS and may decrease the effectiveness of immune-modulating and immune-suppressing medications.

Additional information:

Dosage: variable dosing; 0.5–2.0 g dry ginseng root P.O. daily or 200–600 mg ginseng extract (4% total ginsenoside) P.O. daily

Contraindications and warnings: cardiovascular disease, diabetes, hypertension, hypotension, bleeding disorders, pregnancy, breast-feeding, insomnia, hormone-sensitive cancers and conditions, schizophrenia

Major interactions: anticoagulant and antiplatelet medications, oral hypoglycemic drugs, insulin, steroids, stimulants, immune-suppressing and immune-modulating drugs, MAO inhibitors

Main side effects: insomnia, headache, anxiety, tachycardia, palpitations, hypertension, nausea, vomiting, diarrhea, mastalgia, vaginal bleeding, amenorrhea

References and additional reading:

Bowling AC. *Alternative Medicine and Multiple Sclerosis.* New York: Demos Medical Publishing, Inc., 2001:109–110.

Brinker F. *Herb Contraindications and Drug Interactions.* Sandy, OR: Eclectic Medical Publications, 1998:77.

Ernst E, Pittler MH, Stevinson C, White A. *The Desktop Guide to Complementary and Alternative Medicine: An Evidence-Based Approach.* London: Harcourt Publishers Limited, 2001:87–89.

Fetrow CW, Avila JR. *Professional's Handbook of Complementary & Alternative Medicines.* 2nd ed. Springhouse, PA: Springhouse Corp, 2001:338–342.

Fragakis AS. *The Health Professional's Guide to Popular Dietary Supplements.* 2nd ed. Chicago, IL: American Dietetic Association, 2003:211–221.

Jellin JM, Gregory PJ, Batz F, et al. *Pharmacist's Letter/Prescriber's Letter Natural Medicines Comprehensive Database.* 4th ed. Stockton, CA: Therapeutic Research Faculty, 2002:593–597.

Newall CA, Anderson LA, Phillipson JD. *Herbal Medicines: A Guide for Health-Care Professionals.* London: The Pharmaceutical Press, 1996:145–150.

Scaglione F, Ferrara F, Dugnani, et al. Immunomodulatory effects of two extracts of *Panax ginseng* C.A. Meyer. *Drugs Exp Clin Res* 1990;16:537–542.

Shin JY, Song JY, Yun YS, et al. Immunostimulating effects of acidic polysaccharides extract of *Panax ginseng* on macrophage function. *Immunopharmacol Immunotoxicol*. 2002;24:469–482.

ASTRAGALUS

Other names: Astragali, Beg Kei, Bei Qi, Huang Qi

SUMMARY: Saponins and other polysaccharide components of this herb may stimulate the immune system; this immune-stimulating effect poses theoretical risks in MS and may decrease the effectiveness of immune-modulating and immune-suppressing drugs.

References and additional reading:

Fetrow CW, Avila JR. *Professional's Handbook of Complementary & Alternative Medicines.* 2nd ed. Springhouse, PA: Springhouse Corp, 2001:49–51.

Jellin JM, Gregory PJ, Batz F, et al. *Pharmacist's Letter/Prescriber's Letter Natural Medicines Comprehensive Database.* 4th ed. Stockton, CA: Therapeutic Research Faculty, 2002:103–105.

Peirce A. *Practical Guide to Natural Medicines.* New York: The Stonesong Press, 1999:53–56.

Sun Y, Hersh EM, Lee SL, et al. Preliminary observations on the effects of the Chinese medicinal herbs *Astragalus membranaceus* and *Ligustrum lucidum* on lymphocyte blastogenic responses. *J Biol Resp Mod* 1983;2:227–237.

Zhao KS, Mancini C, Doria G. Enhancement of the immune response in mice by *Astragalus membranaceus* extracts. *Immunopharmacol* 1990;20:225–234.

BARBERRY

Other names: two related herbs are referred to as barberry: (1) Oregon grape—also known as California barberry and trailing mahonia; (2) European barberry—also known as berberis, common barberry, sowberry

SUMMARY: Both types of barberry (as well as goldenseal) contain berberine, a sedating compound that could worsen MS-related fatigue or potentiate the sedating effects of medications. Other side effects include gastrointestinal conditions (nausea, vomiting, diarrhea), nephritis, and spontaneous abortion.

References and additional reading:

Fetrow CW, Avila JR. *Professional's Handbook of Complementary & Alternative Medicines.* 2nd ed. Springhouse, PA: Springhouse Corp, 2001:56–57.

Jellin JM, Gregory PJ, Batz F, et al. *Pharmacist's Letter/Prescriber's Letter Natural Medicines Comprehensive Database.* 4th ed. Stockton, CA: Therapeutic Research Faculty, 2002:948–949.

Peirce A. *Practical Guide to Natural Medicines.* New York: The Stonesong Press, 1999:59–61, 659–661.

BAYBERRY

Other names: candleberry, myrica, sweet oak, tallow shrub, wax myrtle, waxberry

SUMMARY: There is no reliable efficacy data for the oral use of bayberry for any condition. One of the chemical constituents of this herb, a triterpene compound known as myricadiol, has mineralocorticoid effects that may promote salt and water retention and interfere with treatment with steroids as well as antihypertensive medications.

References and additional reading:

Fetrow CW, Avila JR. *Professional's Handbook of Complementary & Alternative Medicines.* 2nd ed. Springhouse, PA: Springhouse Corp, 2001:64–66.

Jellin JM, Gregory PJ, Batz F, et al. *Pharmacist's Letter/Prescriber's Letter Natural Medicines Comprehensive Database.* 4th ed. Stockton, CA: Therapeutic Research Faculty, 2002:115–116.

Newall CA, Anderson LA, Phillipson JD. *Herbal Medicines: A Guide for Health-Care Professionals.* London: The Pharmaceutical Press, 1996:41.

Peirce A. *Practical Guide to Natural Medicines.* New York: The Stonesong Press, 1999:67–69.

BEARBERRY

Other names: arberry, bear's grape, foxberry, mountain cranberry, uva-ursi

SUMMARY: This herb is possibly effective in treating urinary tract infections, but further studies are needed. There is concern about the safety of bearberry, especially for long-term use, because it contains hydroquinone, a chemical with mutagenic and carcinogenic effects.

Additional information:

Dosage: 1–10 g dried herb P.O. daily

Contraindications and warnings: renal disease, gastrointestinal conditions, pregnancy (oxytocic), lactation (insufficient information)

Major interactions: urine acidifiers, including methanamine and vitamin C, may inactivate bearberry; diuretics

Main side effects: green-colored urine, nausea, vomiting, gastrointestinal pain

References and additional reading:

Fetrow CW, Avila JR. *Professional's Handbook of Complementary & Alternative Medicines*. 2nd ed. Springhouse, PA: Springhouse Corp, 2001:66–68.

Jellin JM, Gregory PJ, Batz F, et al. *Pharmacist's Letter/Prescriber's Letter Natural Medicines Comprehensive Database*. 4th ed. Stockton, CA: Therapeutic Research Faculty, 2002:1259–1261.

Newall CA, Anderson LA, Phillipson JD. *Herbal Medicines: A Guide for Health-Care Professionals*. London: The Pharmaceutical Press, 1996:258–259.

Peirce A. *Practical Guide to Natural Medicines*. New York: The Stonesong Press, 1999:647–649.

Schulz V, Hänsel R, Tyler VE. *Rational Phytotherapy: A Physicians' Guide to Herbal Medicine*. 3rd ed. Berlin: Springer-Verlag, 1998:222–224.

BEE POLLEN

Other names: honey bee pollen, pollen

SUMMARY: Although bee pollen is claimed to be effective for many conditions, there is no evidence to support its use for any condition. Rarely, it may cause severe allergic reactions in people with pollen, bee sting, or honey allergies.

References and additional reading:

Bowling AC. *Alternative Medicine and Multiple Sclerosis*. New York: Demos Medical Publishing, Inc., 2001:46–51.

Fetrow CW, Avila JR. *Professional's Handbook of Complementary & Alternative Medicines*. 2nd ed. Springhouse, PA: Springhouse Corp, 2001:68–70.

Fragakis AS. *The Health Professional's Guide to Popular Dietary Supplements*. 2nd ed. Chicago, IL: American Dietetic Association, 2003:33–36.

Jellin JM, Gregory PJ, Batz F, et al. *Pharmacist's Letter/Prescriber's Letter Natural Medicines Comprehensive Database*. 4th ed. Stockton, CA: Therapeutic Research Faculty, 2002:118–119.

BELLADONNA

Other names: deadly nightshade, devil's cherries

SUMMARY: In the United States, belladonna is available as a prescription drug for the treatment of spasms and colic-like pain of the GI tract and bile ducts. Without medical supervision and the use of standardized preparations, belladonna preparations may cause serious anticholinergic side effects. Belladonna may worsen the anticholinergic side effects of prescription medications, including amantadine, tricyclic antidepressants, and others (antihistamines, atropine, hyoscyamine, phenothiazines, quinidine, scopolamine).

References and additional reading:

Ernst E, Pittler MH, Stevinson C, White A. *The Desktop Guide to Complementary and Alternative Medicine: An Evidence-Based Approach.* London: Harcourt Publishers Limited, 2001:69–70.

Jellin JM, Gregory PJ, Batz F, et al. *Pharmacist's Letter/Prescriber's Letter Natural Medicines Comprehensive Database.* 4th ed. Stockton, CA: Therapeutic Research Faculty, 202:126–128.

BETA-CAROTENE: see "vitamin A"

BISSY NUT: see "cola nut"

BLACK COHOSH

Other names: black snakeroot, bugbane, cimicifuga, phytoestrogen, rattleweed, squawroot

SUMMARY: Black cohosh, which is possibly effective for treating menopause symptoms, contains salicylates that may increase the toxicity of methotrexate and may increase the risk of bleeding when taken concomitantly with antiplatelet or anticoagulant medications.

References and additional reading:

Brinker F. *Herb Contraindications and Drug Interactions.* Sandy, OR: Eclectic Medical Publications, 1998:146.

Ernst E, Pittler MH, Stevinson C, White A. *The Desktop Guide to Complementary and Alternative Medicine: An Evidence-Based Approach.* London: Harcourt Publishers Limited, 2001:89–91.

Jellin JM, Gregory PJ, Batz F, et al. *Pharmacist's Letter/Prescriber's Letter Natural Medicines Comprehensive Database.* 4th ed. Stockton, CA: Therapeutic Research Faculty, 2002:161–163.

Newall CA, Anderson LA, Phillipson JD. *Herbal Medicines: A Guide for Health-Care Professionals.* London: The Pharmaceutical Press, 1996:80–81, 280.

BLACK CURRANT SEED OIL

Other names: European black currant, cassis

SUMMARY: Like evening primrose and borage seed oils, black currant seed oil contains relatively high levels (14–19%) of gamma-linolenic acid (GLA), an omega-six polyunsaturated fatty acid (PUFA). Supplementing the diet with linoleic acid, another omega-six fatty acid, may mildly decrease relapse severity and disease progression in MS (see Appendix I). There is limited information about the safety of black currant seed oil, especially for long-term use. Evening primrose oil may be a safer source of GLA than black currant seed oil. If supplements of black currant seed oil or other PUFAs are consumed on a regular basis, vitamin E supplements (0.6–0.9 IU of vitamin E/g PUFA) should be taken to prevent vitamin E deficiency. Patients should be told that this approach should not be used *instead of* disease-modifying medications and that the effects of "combination treatment" with omega-6 PUFAs and disease-modifying medications in MS have not been studied.

Additional information:

Dosage: 500–1000 mg P.O. daily; GLA doses up to 2800 mg daily appear to be well tolerated

Contraindications and warnings: for other GLA-containing oils: epilepsy or schizophrenia (increased risk of seizures), bleeding disorders (prolonged bleeding time), pregnancy and lactation (insufficient information)

Major interactions: for other GLA-containing oils: phenothiazines and other epileptogenic medications (decreased seizure threshold), anticonvulsants, anticoagulant and antiplatelet medications

Main side effects: limited safety information is available, especially for long-term use; GLA-containing oils may cause seizures, gastrointestinal symptoms (nausea, vomiting, soft stools, belching, bloating), bleeding, and bruising; since supplementation with PUFAs may produce vitamin E deficiency, supplementation with vitamin E may be necessary (0.6–0.9 IU of vitamin E/g PUFA)

References and additional reading:

Bates D, Fawcett P, Shaw D, et al. Polyunsaturated fatty acids in treatment of acute remitting multiple sclerosis. *Br Med J* 1978;2:1390–1391.

Bowling AC. *Alternative Medicine and Multiple Sclerosis.* New York: Demos Medical Publishing, Inc., 2001:74–90.

Bowling AC, Stewart TM. Current complementary and alternative therapies for multiple sclerosis. *Curr Treat Options Neurol* 2003;5:55–68.

Dworkin R, Bates D, Millar J, et al. Linoleic acid and multiple sclerosis: a reanalysis of three double-blind trials. *Neurol* 1984;34:1441–1445.

Fragakis AS. *The Health Professional's Guide to Popular Dietary Supplements*. 2nd ed. Chicago, IL: American Dietetic Association, 2003:180–191.

Jellin JM, Gregory PJ, Batz F, et al. *Pharmacist's Letter/Prescriber's Letter Natural Medicines Comprehensive Database*. 4th ed. Stockton, CA: Therapeutic Research Faculty, 2002:165–166, 517–519.

Millar J, Zilkha K, Langman M, et al. Double-blind trial of linoleate supplementation of the diet in multiple sclerosis. *Br Med J* 1973;1:765–768.

Paty D. Double-blind trial of linoleic acid in multiple sclerosis. *Arch Neurol* 1983;40:693–694.

Peirce A. *Practical Guide to Natural Medicines*. New York: The Stonesong Press, 1999:88–90.

BLUE-GREEN ALGAE: see "spirulina"

BONESET

Other names: agueweed, crosswort, eupatorium, feverwort, sweating plant

SUMMARY: Due to its immune-stimulating effects, boneset poses theoretical risks in MS and may antagonize the effects of immune-modulating and immune-suppressing medications. Boneset may contain hepatotoxic pyrrolizidine alkaloids.

References and additional reading:

Fetrow CW, Avila JR. *Professional's Handbook of Complementary & Alternative Medicines*. 2nd ed. Springhouse, PA: Springhouse Corp, 2001:113–115.

Jellin JM, Gregory PJ, Batz F, et al. *Pharmacist's Letter/Prescriber's Letter Natural Medicines Comprehensive Database*. 4th ed. Stockton, CA: Therapeutic Research Faculty, 2002:205–206.

Newall CA, Anderson LA, Phillipson JD. *Herbal Medicines: A Guide for Health-Care Professionals*. London: The Pharmaceutical Press, 1996:48.

Peirce A. *Practical Guide to Natural Medicines*. New York: The Stonesong Press, 1999:107–110.

BORAGE SEED OIL

Other names: borage oil, common borage, starflower

SUMMARY: Like evening primrose and black currant seed oils, borage seed oil contains a relatively high concentration (20–26%) of gamma-linolenic acid (GLA), an omega-six polyunsaturated fatty acid (PUFA). Supplementation of the diet with linoleic acid, another omega-six fatty acid, may mildly decrease relapse severity and disease progression in MS (see Appendix I). Borage seed oil may contain pyrrolizidine alkaloids, which are hepatotoxic. Consequently, as a source of GLA, evening primrose oil may be safer than borage seed oil. If supplements of black currant seed oil or other PUFAs are consumed on a regular basis, vitamin E supplements (0.6–0.9 IU of vitamin E/g PUFA) should be taken to prevent vitamin E deficiency. Patients should be told that this approach should not be used *instead of* disease-modifying medications and that the effects of "combination treatment" with omega-6 PUFAs and disease-modifying medications in MS have not been studied.

Additional information:

Dosage: 1 g P.O. once or twice daily; GLA doses up to 2800 mg daily appear to be well tolerated

Contraindications and warnings: liver disease (hepatotoxicity); for GLA-containing oils generally, epilepsy or schizophrenia (increased risk of seizures) and bleeding disorders (prolonged bleeding time), pregnancy and lactation (insufficient information)

Major interactions: hepatotoxic medications, including methotrexate and interferons; for GLA-containing oils generally, phenothiazines and other epileptogenic medications (decreased seizure threshold), anticonvulsants, and anticoagulant and antiplatelet medications

Main side effects: possible hepatotoxicity due to pyrrolizidine alkaloids; for GLA-containing oils generally, seizures, gastrointestinal symptoms (nausea, vomiting, loose stools, belching, bloating), bleeding, and bruising; since supplementation with PUFAs may produce vitamin E deficiency, supplementation with vitamin E may be necessary (0.6–0.9 IU of vitamin E/g PUFA)

References and additional reading:

Bates D, Fawcett P, Shaw D, et al. Polyunsaturated fatty acids in treatment of acute remitting multiple sclerosis. *Br Med J* 1978;2:1390–1391.

Dworkin R, Bates D, Millar J, et al. Linoleic acid and multiple sclerosis: a reanalysis of three double-blind trials. *Neurol* 1984;34:1441–1445.

Fetrow CW, Avila JR. *Professional's Handbook of Complementary & Alternative Medicines.* 2nd ed. Springhouse, PA: Springhouse Corp, 2001:115–119.

Fragakis AS. *The Health Professional's Guide to Popular Dietary Supplements.* 2nd ed. Chicago, IL: American Dietetic Association, 2003:180–191.

Jellin JM, Gregory PJ, Batz F, et al. *Pharmacist's Letter/Prescriber's Letter Natural Medicines Comprehensive Database.* 4th ed. Stockton, CA: Therapeutic Research Faculty, 2002:207–209.

Paty D. Double-blind trial of linoleic acid in multiple sclerosis. *Arch Neurol* 1983;40:693–694.

Peirce A. *Practical Guide to Natural Medicines.* New York: The Stonesong Press, 1999:110–112.

Millar J, Zilkha K, Langman M, et al. Double-blind trial of linoleate supplementation of the diet in multiple sclerosis. *Br Med J* 1973;1:765–768.

CAFFEINE

Other names: caffeine citrate

SUMMARY: Caffeine, which is available in tablets, coffee, and other forms (tea, cola, guarana, mate), is likely effective in improving mental alertness and is reported by some MS patients to improve fatigue. Surprisingly, there are not any clinical trials that have formally evaluated its effects on MS-related fatigue. Reasonable doses (up to 250 mg daily) are generally well tolerated, but the diuretic and urinary irritant effects of caffeine may worsen MS-associated bladder difficulties and caffeine use may be a risk factor for osteoporosis, a condition to which MS patients may be especially prone.

Additional information:

Dosage: 250 mg or less daily

Contraindications and warnings: pregnancy and breast-feeding; use with caution, especially in chronic high doses, with cardiac arrhythmias, depression, anxiety, diabetes (hypoglycemia), hypertension, renal disease, bladder dysfunction, peptic ulcer disease, and possibly seizure disorders

Major interactions: increased caffeine serum concentrations with cimetidine (Tagamet), disulfiram (Antabuse), estrogen (Estrace), fluvoxamine (Luvox), mexiletine (Mexitil), oral contraceptives, quinolones, riluzole (Rilutek), terbinafine (Lamisil), verapamil (Calan, Verelan); other interactions are possible, especially in chronic high doses, with benzodiazepines (decreased sedative and anxiolytic effect), clozapine (Clozaril) (worsened psychosis), CNS stimulants (increased CNS adverse effects), oral hypoglycemic drugs and insulin (hyperglycemia), MAOIs (hypertensive crisis), and theophylline (increased theophylline serum concentrations)

Main side effects: FDA-approved and generally well tolerated; possible side effects, especially with chronic high doses, include insomnia, anxiety, gastric irritation, nausea, vomiting, tachycardia, hypertension, tremors, muscle fasciculations, delirium, possibly decreased seizure threshold; chronic use may produce tolerance, habituation, and psychological dependence; abrupt discontinuation may cause withdrawal symptoms, including headaches, anxiety, and dizziness

References and additional reading:

Bowling AC. *Alternative Medicine and Multiple Sclerosis.* New York: Demos Medical Publishing, Inc., 2001:103–105.

Brinker F. *Herb Contraindications and Drug Interactions.* Sandy, OR: Eclectic Medical Publications, 1998:57–60.

Fetrow CW, Avila JR. *Professional's Handbook of Complementary & Alternative Medicines.* 2nd ed. Springhouse, PA: Springhouse Corp, 2001:215–218.

Foster S, Tyler VE. *Tyler's Honest Herbal.* 4th ed. New York: The Haworth Herbal Press, 1999:77–81.

Jellin JM, Gregory PJ, Batz F, et al. *Pharmacist's Letter/Prescriber's Letter Natural Medicines Comprehensive Database.* 4th ed. Stockton, CA: Therapeutic Research Faculty, 2002:245–249.

Weinberg BA, Bealer BK. *The World of Caffeine: The Science and Culture of the World's Most Popular Drug.* New York: Routledge, 2001.

CALCIUM

Other names: bone meal, oyster shell calcium

SUMMARY: Calcium and vitamin D are effective in preventing and treating osteoporosis, a condition that is probably underdiagnosed and undertreated in MS patients. In addition, calcium and vitamin D have mild immunosuppressive effects and decrease the severity of experimental allergic encephalomyelitis (EAE). One uncontrolled study found that attack rate was decreased in 10 MS patients who were treated with supplements of calcium, magnesium, and cod-liver oil (which contains vitamin D as well as omega-3 fatty acids). Preliminary results from a small short-term clinical trial of 19–nor, a vitamin D analog, in MS patients indicate this treatment does not decrease disease activity, as assessed by attack rate and MRI measures. Further clinical trials are needed to determine if calcium and vitamin D have disease-modifying effects in MS.

Additional information:

Dosage: for prevention of osteoporosis, 1000–1600 mg elemental calcium daily; unless otherwise indicated, elemental calcium content is 40% for calcium carbonate, 21% for calcium citrate, 13% for calcium lactate, and 9% for calcium gluconate; Tolerable Upper Intake Level (UL) is 2500 mg elemental calcium daily; dietary reference intakes (DRIs) for elemental calcium are 1000 mg for 19–50 years, 1200 mg for > 50 years, 1300 mg for pregnant or lactating women < 19 years, 1000 mg for pregnant or lactating women ≥ 19 years

Contraindications and warnings: hypoparathyroidism, hyperphosphatemia, renal insufficiency, sarcoidosis

Major interactions: thiazide and thiazide-like diuretics (milk alkali syndrome); absorption of some drugs (bisphosphonates, fluoroquinolones, levothyroxine, tetracyclines) and minerals (iron, zinc, magnesium) may be decreased by concomitant administration with calcium

Main side effects: gastrointestinal irritation; flatulence; belching; daily doses greater than 4000 mg may cause renal insufficiency, hypercalcemia, and ectopic calcium deposition

References and additional reading:

Bowling AC. *Alternative Medicine and Multiple Sclerosis.* New York: Demos Medical Publishing, Inc., 2001:191–193.

Bowling AC, Ibrahim R, Stewart TM. Alternative medicine and multiple sclerosis: an objective review from an American perspective. *Int J MS Care* 2000;2:14–21.

Bowling AC, Stewart TM. Current complementary and alternative therapies for multiple sclerosis. *Curr Treat Options Neurol* 2003;5:55–68.

Fleming J, Hummel A, Beinlich B, et al. Vitamin D treatment of relapsing-remitting multiple sclerosis (RRMS): a MRI-based pilot study. *Neurol* 2000;54:A338.

Fragakis AS. *The Health Professional's Guide to Popular Dietary Supplements.* 2nd ed. Chicago, IL: American Dietetic Association, 2003:58–67.

Goldberg P, Fleming M, Picard H. Multiple sclerosis: decreased relapse rate through dietary supplementation with calcium, magnesium, and vitamin D. *Med Hyp* 1986;21:193–200.

Jellin JM, Gregory PJ, Batz F, et al. *Pharmacist's Letter/Prescriber's Letter Natural Medicines Comprehensive Database.* 4th ed. Stockton, CA: Therapeutic Research Faculty, 2002:253–258.

CALENDULA

Other names: garden marigold, holligold, marigold, pot marigold

SUMMARY: Since this herb may be sedating, it may worsen MS fatigue or potentiate the sedating effects of medications. Also, it contains polysaccharides with immune-stimulating effects; these effects pose theoretical risks in MS and could antagonize the effects of immune-modulating and immune-suppressing medications.

References and additional reading:

Amirghofran Z, Azadbakht M, Karimi MH. Evaluation of the immunomodulatory effects of five herbal plants. *J Ethnopharmacol* 2000:72;167–172.

Duke JA, Bogenschutz-Godwin MJ, duCellier J, Duke P-AK. *Handbook of Medicinal Herbs.* 2nd ed. Boca Raton, FL: CRC Press, 2002:139–140.

Jellin JM, Gregory PJ, Batz F, et al. *Pharmacist's Letter/Prescriber's Letter Natural Medicines Comprehensive Database.* 4th ed. Stockton, CA: Therapeutic Research Faculty, 2002:259–260.

Newall CA, Anderson LA, Phillipson JD. *Herbal Medicines: A Guide for Health-Care Professionals.* London: The Pharmaceutical Press, 1996:58–59.

CALIFORNIA POPPY

Other names: none

SUMMARY: This herb has possible sedating effects that could worsen MS fatigue or potentiate the sedating effects of medications.

References and additional reading:

Jellin JM, Gregory PJ, Batz F, et al. *Pharmacist's Letter/Prescriber's Letter Natural Medicines Comprehensive Database.* 4th ed. Stockton, CA: Therapeutic Research Faculty, 2002:261–262.

CAPSICUM

Other names: capsaicin, cayenne, chili pepper, hot pepper, paprika

SUMMARY: Topical preparations of capsicum are effective and safe for treating some forms of pain, including neuropathic pain. Oral administration, especially in high doses, may cause multiple adverse effects. These adverse effects include sedation that could worsen MS fatigue or potentiate the sedating effects of medications.

References and additional reading:

Jellin JM, Gregory PJ, Batz F, et al. *Pharmacist's Letter/Prescriber's Letter Natural Medicines Comprehensive Database.* 4th ed. Stockton, CA: Therapeutic Research Faculty, 2002:273–275.

CASCARA

Other names: bitter bark, buckthorn, cascara sagrada, dogwood bark, sagrada bark, yellow bark

SUMMARY: This herb, which is FDA-approved as a safe and effective laxative, is usually well tolerated. It may cause hypokalemia when used concomitantly with steroids.

References and additional reading:

Brinker F. *Herb Contraindications and Drug Interactions*. Sandy, OR: Eclectic Medical Publications, 1998:47–49.

Duke JA, Bogenschutz-Godwin MJ, duCellier J, Duke P-AK. *Handbook of Medicinal Herbs*. 2nd ed. Boca Raton, FL: CRC Press, 2002:157–158.

Fetrow CW, Avila JR. *Professional's Handbook of Complementary & Alternative Medicines*. 2nd ed. Springhouse, PA: Springhouse Corp, 2001:155–157.

Jellin JM, Gregory PJ, Batz F, et al. *Pharmacist's Letter/Prescriber's Letter Natural Medicines Comprehensive Database*. 4th ed. Stockton, CA: Therapeutic Research Faculty, 2002:285–286.

Newall CA, Anderson LA, Phillipson JD. *Herbal Medicines: A Guide for Health-Care Professionals*. London: The Pharmaceutical Press, 1996:62.

CATNIP

Other names: catmint, catswort, field balm

SUMMARY: Catnip is sometimes claimed to be effective for treating MS, but there are no studies to support its use in MS and it has sedating properties that could worsen MS fatigue or potentiate the sedating effects of medications.

References and additional reading:

Fetrow CW, Avila JR. *Professional's Handbook of Complementary & Alternative Medicines*. 2nd ed. Springhouse, PA: Springhouse Corp, 2001:160–162.

Jellin JM, Gregory PJ, Batz F, et al. *Pharmacist's Letter/Prescriber's Letter Natural Medicines Comprehensive Database*. 4th ed. Stockton, CA: Therapeutic Research Faculty, 2002:298–300.

CAT'S CLAW

Other names: griffe du chat, life-giving vine of Peru, samento, una de gato

SUMMARY: Cat's claw has multiple immunologic effects. The immune-stimulating alkaloids in the herb pose theoretical risks in MS and may interfere with the effects of immune-modulating or immunosuppressive medications.

References and additional reading:

Fetrow CW, Avila JR. *Professional's Handbook of Complementary & Alternative Medicines.* 2nd ed. Springhouse, PA: Springhouse Corp, 2001:162–165.

Jellin JM, Gregory PJ, Batz F, et al. *Pharmacist's Letter/Prescriber's Letter Natural Medicines Comprehensive Database.* 4th ed. Stockton, CA: Therapeutic Research Faculty, 2002:295–296.

Peirce A. *Practical Guide to Natural Medicines.* New York: The Stonesong Press, 1999:149–150.

Sheng Y, Bryngelsson C, Pero RW. Enhanced DNA repair, immune function, and reduced toxicity of C-MED-100, a novel aqueous extract from *Uncaria tomentosa. J Ethnopharmacol* 2000:69;115–126.

CELANDINE

Other names: chelidonii, common celandine, greater celandine, rock poppy, wart wort

SUMMARY: Use of this herb should be avoided due to multiple possible adverse effects, including hepatitis, coma, and death. In addition, this herb has immune-stimulating effects that pose theoretical risks in MS and may interfere with the effects of immune-modulating and immune-suppressing medications.

References and additional reading:

Duke JA, Bogenschutz-Godwin MJ, duCellier J, Duke P-AK. *Handbook of Medicinal Herbs.* 2nd ed. Boca Raton, FL: CRC Press, 2002:168–169.

Fetrow CW, Avila JR. *Professional's Handbook of Complementary & Alternative Medicines.* 2nd ed. Springhouse, PA: Springhouse Corp, 2001:165–167.

Jellin JM, Gregory PJ, Batz F, et al. *Pharmacist's Letter/Prescriber's Letter Natural Medicines Comprehensive Database.* 4th ed. Stockton, CA: Therapeutic Research Faculty, 2002:639–640.

Nowicky JW, Staniszewski A, Zbroja-Sontag W, et al. Evaluation of thiophosphoric acid alkaloid derivatives from *Chelidonium majus* L. (Ukrain) as an immunostimulant in patients with various carcinomas. *Drugs Exp Clin Res* 1991;17:139–143.

Song JY, Yang HO, Pyo SN, et al. Immunomodulatory activity of protein-bound polysaccharide extracted from *Chelidonium majus. Arch Pharm Res* 2002; 25:158–164.

CELERY

Other names: celery fruit, celery seed, marsh parsley

SUMMARY: Large doses of celery fruit, which is different from the commonly eaten celery stem, have sedating properties that may worsen MS fatigue or potentiate the sedating effects of medications.

References and additional reading:

Fetrow CW, Avila JR. *Professional's Handbook of Complementary & Alternative Medicines*. 2nd ed. Springhouse, PA: Springhouse Corp, 2001:169–171.

Jellin JM, Gregory PJ, Batz F, et al. *Pharmacist's Letter/Prescriber's Letter Natural Medicines Comprehensive Database*. 4th ed. Stockton, CA: Therapeutic Research Faculty, 2002:305–306.

Newall CA, Anderson LA, Phillipson JD. *Herbal Medicines: A Guide for Health-Care Professionals*. London: The Pharmaceutical Press, 1996:65–66.

Peirce A. *Practical Guide to Natural Medicines*. New York: The Stonesong Press, 1999:152–155.

CHAMOMILE

Other names: German chamomile, manzanilla, pin heads, wild chamomile

SUMMARY: Chamomile has sedating properties that may worsen MS fatigue or potentiate the sedating effects of medications.

References and additional reading:

Fetrow CW, Avila JR. *Professional's Handbook of Complementary & Alternative Medicines*. 2nd ed. Springhouse, PA: Springhouse Corp, 2001:173–175.

Jellin JM, Gregory PJ, Batz F, et al. *Pharmacist's Letter/Prescriber's Letter Natural Medicines Comprehensive Database*. 4th ed. Stockton, CA: Therapeutic Research Faculty, 2002:578–579.

Newall CA, Anderson LA, Phillipson JD. *Herbal Medicines: A Guide for Health-Care Professionals*. London: The Pharmaceutical Press, 1996:69–71.

Peirce A. *Practical Guide to Natural Medicines*. New York: The Stonesong Press, 1999:155–158.

CHAPARRAL

Other names: creosote bush, greasewood, hediondilla

SUMMARY: Chaparral is sometimes claimed to be an effective treatment for MS. However, there is no evidence for its efficacy in MS or any other disease, and its use should be avoided due to serious toxicity, including irreversible hepatotoxicity.

References and additional reading:

Brinker F. *Herb Contraindications and Drug Interactions.* Sandy, OR: Eclectic Medical Publications, 1998:54.

Fetrow CW, Avila JR. *Professional's Handbook of Complementary & Alternative Medicines.* 2nd ed. Springhouse, PA: Springhouse Corp, 2001:175–177.

Jellin JM, Gregory PJ, Batz F, et al. *Pharmacist's Letter/Prescriber's Letter Natural Medicines Comprehensive Database.* 4th ed. Stockton, CA: Therapeutic Research Faculty, 2002:311–312.

Peirce A. *Practical Guide to Natural Medicines.* New York: The Stonesong Press, 1999:159–161.

COD LIVER OIL

Other names: cod oil

SUMMARY: Cod-liver oil contains high concentrations of two types of omega-3 polyunsaturated fatty acids (PUFAs), eicosapentanoic acid (EPA) and docosahexanoic acid (DHA). EPA and DHA may also be obtained from fish oil, concentrated preparations of EPA and DHA, and fatty fish, such as salmon, mackerel, sardines, herring, tuna, and bluefish. Omega-3 fatty acids have mild immunosuppressive effects. One large controlled trial of omega-3 fatty acid supplementation in MS patients reported a trend toward benefit (p=0.07). Two uncontrolled studies and one recent preliminary study reported significant benefits of omega-3 fatty acid supplementation in MS patients (see Appendix I). Further studies are needed to determine if omega-3 fatty acids have therapeutic effects in MS. Some MS patients may want to use this approach based on the limited evidence; in this situation, it should be emphasized that reasonable doses ($\leq$3 g combined EPA and DHA intake daily) should be taken, vitamin E supplementation may be necessary (0.6–0.9 IU of vitamin E/g PUFA), this approach should not be used *instead of* disease-modifying medications, and the effects of combination treatment with omega-3 fatty acids and disease-modifying medications in MS have not been well studied.

Additional information:

Dosage: in MS clinical trials, the combined daily intake of EPA and DHA has been 0.9–2.85 g; one study used approximately 20 g cod liver oil daily

Contraindications and warnings: bleeding disorders; aspirin sensitivity (decreased pulmonary function); diabetes (high doses may cause hyperglycemia); bipolar disorder and depression (hypomania); pregnancy and lactation (insufficient information)

Major interactions: anticoagulant and antiplatelet medications, oral hypoglycemic medications and insulin (hyperglycemia), antihypertensive medications (hypotension)

Main side effects: generally well tolerated; combined daily intake of EPA
and DHA of 3 g or less has been given the "Generally Regarded as Safe"
(GRAS) designation by the FDA; fishy taste; belching; halitosis; nosebleeds;
bruising; heartburn; high doses may cause nausea and loose stools; cod liver
oil may contain relatively high levels of vitamin A (approximately 15,000 IU
of vitamin A/20 g cod liver oil) and vitamin D (approximately 1500 IU of
vitamin D/20 g cod liver oil) and excessive doses of these vitamins (greater
than 10,000 IU of vitamin A or greater than 2000 IU of vitamin D daily)
should be avoided, especially with vitamin A during pregnancy; since supplementation with PUFAs may produce vitamin E deficiency, supplementation with vitamin E may be necessary (0.6–0.9 IU of vitamin E/g PUFA)

References and additional reading:

Bates D, Cartlidge N, French J, et al. A double-blind controlled trial of long chain
n-3 polyunsaturated fatty acids in the treatment of multiple sclerosis. *J
Neurol Neurosurg Psych* 1989;52:18–22.

Bowling AC. *Alternative Medicine and Multiple Sclerosis.* New York: Demos Medical
Publishing, Inc., 2001:74–90.

Bowling AC, Stewart TM. Current complementary and alternative therapies for
multiple sclerosis. *Curr Treat Options Neurol* 2003;5:55–68.

Fragakis AS. *The Health Professional's Guide to Popular Dietary Supplements.* 2nd ed.
Chicago, IL: American Dietetic Association, 2003:147–160.

Goldberg P, Fleming M, Picard H. Multiple sclerosis: decreased relapse rate through
dietary supplementation with calcium, magnesium and vitamin D. *Med Hyp*
1986;21:193–200.

Jellin JM, Gregory PJ, Batz F, et al. *Pharmacist's Letter/Prescriber's Letter Natural
Medicines Comprehensive Database.* 4th ed. Stockton, CA: Therapeutic
Research Faculty, 2002:368–369.

Nordvik I, Myhr K-M, Nyland H, et al. Effect of dietary advice and n-3 supplementation in newly diagnosed MS patients. *Acta Neurol Scand* 2000;102:143–149.

Weinstock-Guttman B, Baier M, Peterken L, et al. A randomized study of low-fat
diet with w-3 fatty acid supplementation in patients with relapsing-remitting
multiple sclerosis (RRMS). *Neurol* 2002;58:A461–2.

COENZYME Q10

Other names: CoQ, CoQ10, Q10, ubiquinone

SUMMARY: Coenzyme Q10 (CoQ10) is an antioxidant and a cofactor in the
production of ATP. These two functions may give it neuroprotective effects

that could be beneficial in MS. However, like most antioxidants, CoQ10 has immune-stimulating effects that raise theoretical risks in MS and could antagonize the effects of immune-modulating and immune-suppressing medications. High doses of CoQ10 (>300 mg P.O. daily) may cause mild liver toxicity; this effect could increase the potential hepatotoxic effects of medications, including interferons and methotrexate. Further studies are needed to determine the effects, if any, of CoQ10 and other antioxidants in MS. Until more information is available, it may be most reasonable for MS patients to obtain antioxidant compounds through dietary sources such as fruits (two to four servings daily) and vegetables (three to five servings daily). If antioxidant supplements are taken in MS, it may be best to avoid long-term use of high doses or large numbers of different antioxidants.

Additional information:

Dosage: in studies of cardiac disease, 50–300 mg daily

Contraindications and warnings: diabetes (hypoglycemia), pregnancy and lactation (insufficient information)

Major interactions: anticoagulant medications (procoagulant, vitamin K-like effect); oral hypoglycemic medications and insulin; antihypertensive medications (hypotension)

Main side effects: generally well tolerated; nausea; diarrhea; abdominal pain; ischemic tissue damage with intense exercise; high doses (>300 g daily) may increase liver function tests

References and additional reading:

Bowling AC. *Alternative Medicine and Multiple Sclerosis.* New York: Demos Medical Publishing, Inc., 2001:188–190;201.

Bowling AC, Stewart TM. Current complementary and alternative therapies for multiple sclerosis. *Curr Treat Options Neurol* 2003;5:55–68.

Ernst E, Pittler MH, Stevinson C, White A. *The Desktop Guide to Complementary and Alternative Medicine: An Evidence-Based Approach.* London: Harcourt Publishers Limited, 2001:96–98.

Fetrow CW, Avila JR. *Professional's Handbook of Complementary & Alternative Medicines.* 2nd ed. Springhouse, PA: Springhouse Corp, 2001:211–215.

Folkers K, Hanioka T, Xia LJ, et al. Coenzyme Q10 increases T4/T8 ratios of lymphocytes in ordinary subjects and relevance to patients having the AIDS related complex. *Biochem Biophys Res Commun* 1991;176:786–791.

Folkers K, Morita M, McRee J. The activities of coenzyme Q10 and vitamin B6 for immune responses. *Biochem Biophys Res Commun* 1993;193:88–92.

Fragakis AS. *The Health Professional's Guide to Popular Dietary Supplements.* 2nd ed. Chicago, IL: American Dietetic Association, 2003: 94–102.

Jellin JM, Gregory PJ, Batz F, et al. *Pharmacist's Letter/Prescriber's Letter Natural Medicines Comprehensive Database*. 4th ed. Stockton, CA: Therapeutic Research Faculty, 2002:370–373.

COFFEE

Other names: bean juice, café, espresso, java

SUMMARY: Coffee contains 1–2.6% caffeine, the primary active constituent, as well as other active ingredients, including chlorogenic acid, caffeol, and diterpenes. The caffeine content of a cup of coffee is 100–150 mg for percolated coffee, 85–100 mg for instant coffee, and approximately 8 mg for decaffeinated coffee. While caffeine is effective for increasing mental alertness and some MS patients report that caffeine improves fatigue, there are not any studies of the effects of caffeine or coffee on MS fatigue, MS-associated cognitive dysfunction, or other MS-related symptoms. Reasonable doses (up to two to three cups of coffee or 250–300 mg caffeine daily) are usually well tolerated. However, the diuretic and urinary irritant actions of caffeine may provoke MS-associated bladder difficulties and caffeine consumption may increase the risk for osteoporosis, a condition to which MS patients may be particularly susceptible. For additional information, see listing under caffeine.

References and additional reading:

Bowling AC. *Alternative Medicine and Multiple Sclerosis*. New York: Demos Medical Publishing, Inc., 2001:103–105.

Brinker F. *Herb Contraindications and Drug Interactions*. Sandy, OR: Eclectic Medical Publications, 1998:57–60.

Fetrow CW, Avila JR. *Professional's Handbook of Complementary & Alternative Medicines*. 2nd ed. Springhouse, PA: Springhouse Corp, 2001:215–218.

Foster S, Tyler VE. *Tyler's Honest Herbal*. 4th ed. New York: The Haworth Herbal Press, 1999:77–81.

Jellin JM, Gregory PJ, Batz F, et al. *Pharmacist's Letter/Prescriber's Letter Natural Medicines Comprehensive Database*. 4th ed. Stockton, CA: Therapeutic Research Faculty, 2002:245–249, 373–377.

Weinberg BA, Bealer BK. *The World of Caffeine: The Science and Culture of the World's Most Popular Drug*. New York: Routledge, 2001.

COLA NUT

Other names: bissy nut, bissy tea, cola seed, guru nut, kola nut

SUMMARY: Although "bissy tea," which is prepared from the cola nut, is sometimes specifically marketed for MS, there are not any published studies of cola nut use in MS. Caffeine is the active constituent in cola nut. Cola nut typically contains 1–3.5% caffeine. Caffeine improves mental alertness, but it has not been studied as a therapy for MS fatigue or other MS-associated symptoms. In reasonable doses, cola nut is usually well tolerated and has been given "Generally Regarded as Safe" (GRAS) status by the FDA. Cola nut, like coffee and other caffeine-containing herbs, may provoke MS-related bladder dysfunction through the diuretic and urinary irritant actions of caffeine. Also, caffeine consumption may increase the risk for osteoporosis, a condition to which MS patients may be particularly prone. Adverse effects and contraindications that are specific to cola nut are that chewing the nut increases the risk of developing oral cancer, the high tannin content may cause hepatotoxicity (which could be provoked by methotrexate or interferon use in MS), and cross-sensitivity reactions may occur in people who are allergic to chocolate. The usual doses of cola nut are 1–2 g of powdered nut three times daily, one cup of tea three times daily, 0.6–1.2 mL of liquid extract daily, or 1–4 mL tincture of cola nut daily. For additional information, see listing under caffeine.

References and additional reading:

Bowling AC. *Alternative Medicine and Multiple Sclerosis.* New York: Demos Medical Publishing, Inc., 2001:103–105.

Brinker F. *Herb Contraindications and Drug Interactions.* Sandy, OR: Eclectic Medical Publications, 1998:57–62.

Fetrow CW, Avila JR. *Professional's Handbook of Complementary & Alternative Medicines.* 2nd ed. Springhouse, PA: Springhouse Corp, 2001:218–221.

Foster S, Tyler VE. *Tyler's Honest Herbal.* 4th ed. New York: The Haworth Herbal Press, 1999:77–81.

Jellin JM, Gregory PJ, Batz F, et al. *Pharmacist's Letter/Prescriber's Letter Natural Medicines Comprehensive Database.* 4th ed. Stockton, CA: Therapeutic Research Faculty, 2002:245–249, 378–381.

Newall CA, Anderson LA, Phillipson JD. *Herbal Medicines: A Guide for Health-Care Professionals.* London: The Pharmaceutical Press, 1996:84.

Weinberg BA, Bealer BK. *The World of Caffeine: The Science and Culture of the World's Most Popular Drug.* New York: Routledge, 2001.

COMFREY

Other names: ass ear, black root, bruisewort, gum plant, healing herb, knitback, salsify, slippery root, wallwort

SUMMARY: Comfrey is sometimes claimed to be an effective therapy for MS. However, this herb should not be consumed because it contains pyrrolizidine alkaloids, hepatotoxic and hepatocarcinogenic compounds that may cause hepatic veno-occlusive disease.

References and additional reading:

Brinker F. *Herb Contraindications and Drug Interactions.* Sandy, OR: Eclectic Medical Publications, 1998:63.

Fetrow CW, Avila JR. *Professional's Handbook of Complementary & Alternative Medicines.* 2nd ed. Springhouse, PA: Springhouse Corp, 2001:226–229.

Jellin JM, Gregory PJ, Batz F, et al. *Pharmacist's Letter/ Prescriber's Letter Natural Medicines Comprehensive Database.* 4th ed. Stockton, CA: Therapeutic Research Faculty, 2002:388–389.

Newall CA, Anderson LA, Phillipson JD. *Herbal Medicines: A Guide for Health-Care Professionals.* London: The Pharmaceutical Press, 1996:87–89.

COUCH GRASS

Other names: dog grass, durfa grass, quack grass, scotch quelch

SUMMARY: This herb has sedating properties that could worsen MS-associated fatigue or increase the sedating effects of medications.

References and additional reading:

Fetrow CW, Avila JR. *Professional's Handbook of Complementary & Alternative Medicines.* 2nd ed. Springhouse, PA: Springhouse Corp, 2001:236–238.

Jellin JM, Gregory PJ, Batz F, et al. *Pharmacist's Letter/Prescriber's Letter Natural Medicines Comprehensive Database.* 4th ed. Stockton, CA: Therapeutic Research Faculty, 2002:412–413.

Newall CA, Anderson LA, Phillipson JD. *Herbal Medicines: A Guide for Health-Care Professionals.* London: The Pharmaceutical Press, 1996:91.

CRANBERRY

Other names: bog cranberry, trailing swamp cranberry

SUMMARY: Cranberry is possibly effective for preventing urinary tract infections (UTIs). Due to the availability of effective antibiotics and the complications that may occur with an untreated UTI (especially in MS patients), this herb should not be used to treat known infections. Two chemical constituents, proanthocyanidins and fructose, may decrease bacterial adherence to urinary tract epithelial cells. Also, fructose may have antibacterial properties. Although vitamin C or bearberry are also sometimes suggested for UTI prevention, there is more evidence supporting the use of cranberry than these other therapies.

Additional information:

Dosage: optimal dosing has not been established; 1–10 oz juice P.O. daily is sometimes used; six capsules of dried powder or 1.5 oz of fresh or frozen cranberries may be equivalent to 3 oz of juice; capsules are often taken in doses of 300–400 mg P.O. twice daily; cranberry juice cocktail is 26–33% cranberry juice

Contraindications and warnings: nephrolithiasis (possible increased risk of kidney stones due to high oxalate concentration in juice), pregnancy and lactation (insufficient information)

Major interactions: none

Main side effects: chronic use of high doses (greater than 1 L daily) may increase the risk of kidney stone formation and cause gastrointestinal upset and diarrhea

References and additional reading:

Bowling AC. *Alternative Medicine and Multiple Sclerosis.* New York: Demos Medical Publishing, Inc., 2001:105–106.

Fetrow CW, Avila JR. *Professional's Handbook of Complementary & Alternative Medicines.* 2nd ed. Springhouse, PA: Springhouse Corp, 2001:240–243.

Fragakis AS. *The Health Professional's Guide to Popular Dietary Supplements.* 2nd ed. Chicago, IL: American Dietetic Association, 2003: 115–119.

Jellin JM, Gregory PJ, Batz F, et al. *Pharmacist's Letter/Prescriber's Letter Natural Medicines Comprehensive Database.* 4th ed. Stockton, CA: Therapeutic Research Faculty, 2002:421–422.

Peirce A. *Practical Guide to Natural Medicines.* New York: The Stonesong Press, 1999:209–211.

CREATINE

Other names: creatine monohydrate

SUMMARY: Creatine may increase muscle strength in some situations, especially brief, high-intensity exercise. It is being studied in neuromuscular diseases. Also, creatine may have neuroprotective effects and, consequently, is being studied in several different neurodegenerative diseases. In MS, it is theoretically possible that creatine supplements could increase muscle strength or exercise tolerance and slow disease progression, but studies in this area have not been reported.

Additional information:

Dosage: for improving physical performance, loading dose of 20 g (or 0.3 g/kg) P.O. daily for 2–5 days and then maintenance dose of 2 or more g (or 0.03 g/kg) P.O. daily

Contraindications and warnings: renal disease could be worsened by creatine; pregnancy and lactation (insufficient information).

Major interactions: possible potentiation of the nephrotoxic effects of medications

Main side effects: gastrointestinal pain, nausea, diarrhea; dehydration; weight gain; muscle cramping; renal insufficiency, especially with pre-existing renal disease

References and additional reading:

Bowling AC. *Alternative Medicine and Multiple Sclerosis.* New York: Demos Medical Publishing, Inc., 2001:202.

Fetrow CW, Avila JR. *Professional's Handbook of Complementary & Alternative Medicines.* 2nd ed. Springhouse, PA: Springhouse Corp, 2001:244–247.

Fragakis AS. *The Health Professional's Guide to Popular Dietary Supplements.* 2nd ed. Chicago, IL: American Dietetic Association, 2003:119–129.

Jellin JM, Gregory PJ, Batz F, et al. *Pharmacist's Letter/Prescriber's Letter Natural Medicines Comprehensive Database.* 4th ed. Stockton, CA: Therapeutic Research Faculty, 2002:423–425.

Schneider-Gold C, Beck M, Wessig C, et al. Creatine monohydrate in DM2/PROMM. *Neurol* 2003;60:500–502.

Tarnopolsky MA, Beal MF. Potential for creatine and other therapies targeting cellular energy dysfunction in neurological disorders. *Ann Neurol* 2001;49:561–574.

DEHYDROEPIANDROSTERONE: see "DHEA"

DHA: see "fish oil"

DHEA

Other names: dehydroepiandrosterone, prasterone

SUMMARY: This dietary supplement is a hormone that is sometimes claimed to be effective for treating MS. In some studies, it has been shown to exert anti-inflammatory effects and decrease the severity of experimental allergic encephalomyelitis (EAE). However, in other studies, it appears to activate T cells, an effect that poses theoretical risks in MS and may antagonize the actions of immune-modulating and immune-suppressing medications. Further studies are needed to clarify its immunologic actions and its effects, if any, on MS. DHEA may cause hepatic dysfunction and may increase the hepatotoxicity of medications, including methotrexate and interferons. Other adverse effects include acne, hair loss, hirsutism, voice deepening, fatigue, mania, increased risk of hormone-sensitive cancers (breast, endometrial, prostate), insulin resistance, decreased HDL cholesterol, altered menstrual pattern, abdominal pain, and hypertension.

References and additional reading:

Bowling AC. *Alternative Medicine and Multiple Sclerosis*. New York: Demos Medical Publishing, Inc., 2001:202–203.

Du C, Khalil MW, Sriram S. Administration of dehydroepiandrosterone suppresses allergic encephalomyelitis in SJL/J mice. *J Neuroimmunol* 2001;167:7094–7101.

Fetrow CW, Avila JR. *Professional's Handbook of Complementary & Alternative Medicines*. 2nd ed. Springhouse, PA: Springhouse Corp, 2001:263–266.

Fragakis AS. *The Health Professional's Guide to Popular Dietary Supplements*. 2nd ed. Chicago, IL: American Dietetic Association, 2003: 129–138.

Jellin JM, Gregory PJ, Batz F, et al. *Pharmacist's Letter/Prescriber's Letter Natural Medicines Comprehensive Database*. 4th ed. Stockton, CA: Therapeutic Research Faculty, 2002:451–454.

Khorram O, Vu L, Yen SS. Activation of immune function by dehydroepiandrosterone (DHEA) in age-advanced men. *J Gerontol A Biol Sci Med Sci* 1997;52:M1–M7.

Suzuki T, Suzuki N, Daynes RA, et al. Dehydroepiandrosterone enhances IL2 production and cytotoxic effector function of human T cells. *Clin Immunol Immunopathol* 1991;61;202–211.

DOCOSAHEXANOIC ACID (DHA): see "fish oil"

DONG QUAI

Other names: Chinese angelica, tang kuei, women's ginseng

SUMMARY: This Asian herb has immune-stimulating effects that pose theoretical risks in MS and may decrease the effectiveness of immune-modulating and immune-suppressing medications.

References and additional reading:

Fetrow CW, Avila JR. *Professional's Handbook of Complementary & Alternative Medicines*. 2nd ed. Springhouse, PA: Springhouse Corp, 2001:272–274.

Jellin JM, Gregory PJ, Batz F, et al. *Pharmacist's Letter/Prescriber's Letter Natural Medicines Comprehensive Database.* 4th ed. Stockton, CA: Therapeutic Research Faculty, 2002:469–471.

Wilasrusmee C, Siddiqui J, Bruch D, et al. In vitro immunomodulatory effects of herbal products. *Am Surg* 2002;68:860–864.

ECHINACEA

Other names: American coneflower, black Sampson, black Susan, comb flower, coneflower, Indian head, Kansas snakeroot, purple coneflower, Sampson root, scurvy root

SUMMARY: Echinacea is possibly effective in decreasing the duration and severity of the common cold. Since viral infections may cause MS exacerbations, it is theoretically possible that echinacea could decrease the risk of an exacerbation. However, various echinacea constituents, including high molecular weight polysaccharides, alkylamides, and caffeic acid derivatives, stimulate macrophages and T cells. This immune-stimulating effect of echinacea poses theoretical risks in MS and may interfere with the actions of immune-suppressing and immune-modulating medications. There is a case report of a patient who developed acute disseminated encephalomyelitis (ADEM) after intramuscular treatment with a herbal mixture that included echinacea. An additional concern with echinacea is that if it is taken with methotrexate, interferons, or other potentially hepatotoxic medications, there may be an increased risk of hepatotoxicity.

References and additional reading:

Bowling AC. *Alternative Medicine and Multiple Sclerosis.* New York: Demos Medical Publishing, Inc., 2001:106–107.

Ernst E, Pittler MH, Stevinson C, White A. *The Desktop Guide to Complementary and Alternative Medicine: An Evidence-Based Approach.* London: Harcourt Publishers Limited, 2001:102–103.

Fetrow CW, Avila JR. *Professional's Handbook of Complementary & Alternative Medicines.* 2nd ed. Springhouse, PA: Springhouse Corp, 2001:275–278.

Fragakis AS. *The Health Professional's Guide to Popular Dietary Supplements.* 2nd ed. Chicago, IL: American Dietetic Association, 2003:141–146.

Jellin JM, Gregory PJ, Batz F, et al. *Pharmacist's Letter/Prescriber's Letter Natural Medicines Comprehensive Database.* 4th ed. Stockton, CA: Therapeutic Research Faculty, 2002:477–480.

Peirce A. *Practical Guide to Natural Medicines.* New York: The Stonesong Press, 1999:236–239.

Percival SS. Use of echinacea in medicine. *Biochem Pharmacol* 2000;60:155–158.

Schwarz S, Knauth M, Schwab S, et al. Acute disseminated encephalomyelitis after parenteral therapy with herbal extracts: a report of two cases. *J Neurol Neurosurg Psych* 2000;69:516–518.

Vickers A, Zollman C. ABC of complementary medicine: herbal medicine. *Br Med J* 1999;319:10501053.

EICOSAPENTANOIC ACID (EPA): see "fish oil"

EPA: see "fish oil"

ELECAMPANE

Other names: alant, aunee, elfdock, elfwort, horseheal, inula, scabwort, velvet dock, wild sunflower, yellow starwort

SUMMARY: This herb, especially in high doses, has sedative properties that may worsen MS fatigue or increase the sedating effects of medications.

References and additional reading:

Fetrow CW, Avila JR. *Professional's Handbook of Complementary & Alternative Medicines.* 2nd ed. Springhouse, PA: Springhouse Corp, 2001:281–283.

Jellin JM, Gregory PJ, Batz F, et al. *Pharmacist's Letter/Prescriber's Letter Natural Medicines Comprehensive Database.* 4th ed. Stockton, CA: Therapeutic Research Faculty, 2002:486–487.

EPHEDRA

Other names: brigham tea, desert herb, herbal ecstasy, joint fir, ma huang, popotillo, sea grape, yellow astringent

SUMMARY: This herb, which is sometimes marketed for its fatigue-relieving effects, should not be used because of multiple possible toxic effects, including hypertension, cardiac arrhythmias, myocardial infarction, seizures, stroke, and death. The risk of these toxic effects may be increased when ephedra is taken concomitantly with medications, herbs, or other dietary supplements with stimulant effects. Ephedra may decrease the effectiveness of dexamethasone (Decadron®) because ephedrine, the primary active constituent in ephedra, may increase the clearance rate of dexamethasone.

References and additional reading:

Brinker F. *Herb Contraindications and Drug Interactions.* Sandy, OR: Eclectic Medical Publications, 1998:95–97.

Fetrow CW, Avila JR. *Professional's Handbook of Complementary & Alternative Medicines.* 2nd ed. Springhouse, PA: Springhouse Corp, 2001:284–287.

Jellin JM, Gregory PJ, Batz F, et al. *Pharmacist's Letter/Prescriber's Letter Natural Medicines Comprehensive Database.* 4th ed. Stockton, CA: Therapeutic Research Faculty, 2002:497–500.

Peirce A. *Practical Guide to Natural Medicines.* New York: The Stonesong Press, 1999:246–248.

EVENING PRIMROSE OIL

Other names: EPO, fever plant, king's cureall, night willow-herb, primrose, sun drop

SUMMARY: Evening primrose oil (EPO), like black currant and borage seed oils, has a relatively high concentration (2–16%) of gamma-linolenic acid (GLA), an omega-six polyunsaturated fatty acid (PUFA). It also contains 65–80% linoleic acid (another omega-six PUFA), 2–16% oleic acid, 7% palmitic acid, and 3% stearic acid. Although EPO has not shown therapeutic effects in limited clinical trials in relapsing-remitting or progressive MS, controlled clinical trials indicate that linoleic acid supplementation may mildly decrease relapse severity and disease progression in relapsing-remitting MS (see Appendix I). As a source of GLA, evening primrose oil may be safer than black currant or borage seed oils. If supplements of EPO or other PUFAs are consumed on a regular basis, vitamin E supplements (0.6–0.9 IU of vitamin E/gm PUFA) should be taken to prevent vitamin E deficiency. Patients should be told that this approach should not be used *instead of* disease-modifying medications and that the effects of "combination treatment" with omega-6 PUFAs and disease-modifying medications in MS have not been studied.

Additional information:

Dosage: in MS clinical trials, EPO was used at doses that provided 340–360 mg GLA daily; for other diseases, EPO daily doses are usually 2–4 g, 10% of which is GLA; EPO preparations may contain variable concentrations of GLA; GLA doses up to 2800 mg daily appear to be well tolerated

Contraindications and warnings: epilepsy or schizophrenia (increased risk of seizures) and bleeding disorders (prolonged bleeding time), pregnancy (possible increased risk of multiple complications)

Major interactions: for GLA-containing oils generally: phenothiazines and other epileptogenic medications (decreased seizure threshold), anticonvulsants, and anticoagulant and antiplatelet medications

Main side effects: seizures, gastrointestinal symptoms (nausea, vomiting, loose stools, belching, bloating), bleeding, and bruising; since supplementation with PUFAs may produce vitamin E deficiency, supplementation with vitamin E may be necessary (0.6–0.9 IU of vitamin E/g PUFA)

References and additional reading:

Bates D, Fawcett P, Shaw D, et al. Polyunsaturated fatty acids in treatment of acute remitting multiple sclerosis. *Br Med J* 1978;2:1390–1391.

Bates D, Fawcett P, Shaw D, et al. Trial of polyunsaturated fatty acids in non-relapsing multiple sclerosis. *Br Med J* 1977;2:932–933.

Bowling AC. *Alternative Medicine and Multiple Sclerosis.* New York: Demos Medical Publishing, Inc., 2001:74–90.

Bowling AC, Stewart TM. Current complementary and alternative therapies for multiple sclerosis. *Curr Treat Options Neurol* 2003, 5:55–68.

Dworkin R, Bates D, Millar J, et al. Linoleic acid and multiple sclerosis: a reanalysis of three double-blind trials. *Neurol* 1984;34:1441–1445.

Ernst E, Pittler MH, Stevinson C, White A. *The Desktop Guide to Complementary and Alternative Medicine: An Evidence-Based Approach.* London: Harcourt Publishers Limited, 2001:103–106.

Fetrow CW, Avila JR. *Professional's Handbook of Complementary & Alternative Medicines.* 2nd ed. Springhouse, PA: Springhouse Corp, 2001:624–626.

Fragakis AS. *The Health Professional's Guide to Popular Dietary Supplements.* 2nd ed. Chicago, IL: American Dietetic Association, 2003: 180–191.

Jellin JM, Gregory PJ, Batz F, et al. *Pharmacist's Letter/Prescriber's Letter Natural Medicines Comprehensive Database.* 4th ed. Stockton, CA: Therapeutic Research Faculty, 2002:517–519.

Millar J, Zilkha K, Langman M, et al. Double-blind trial of linoleate supplementation of the diet in multiple sclerosis. *Br Med J* 1973;1:765–768.

Paty D. Double-blind trial of linoleic acid in multiple sclerosis. *Arch Neurol* 1983;40:693–694.

FENUGREEK

Other names: bird's foot, Greek hay, trigonella

SUMMARY: Fenugreek may decrease the effectiveness of steroid medications.

References and additional reading:

Fetrow CW, Avila JR. *Professional's Handbook of Complementary & Alternative Medicines.* 2nd ed. Springhouse, PA: Springhouse Corp, 2001:296–299.

Jellin JM, Gregory PJ, Batz F, et al. *Pharmacist's Letter/Prescriber's Letter Natural Medicines Comprehensive Database.* 4th ed. Stockton, CA: Therapeutic Research Faculty, 2002:524–526.

Newall CA, Anderson LA, Phillipson JD. *Herbal Medicines: A Guide for Health-Care Professionals.* London: The Pharmaceutical Press, 1996:117–118.

FISH OIL

Other names: fish body oil, fish oil fatty acids, Menhaden oil

SUMMARY: Fish oil contains high concentrations of eicosapentanoic acid (EPA) and docosahexanoic acid (DHA), two types of omega-3 polyunsaturated fatty acids (PUFAs). Fish oil supplements typically contain 180–300 mg EPA and 120–200 mg DHA per capsule. EPA and DHA may also be obtained from cod liver oil, concentrated preparations of EPA and DHA, and fatty fish, such as salmon, mackerel, sardines, herring, tuna, and bluefish. Omega-3 PUFAs have mild immunosuppressive effects. A large controlled trial of omega-3 PUFA supplementation in MS patients found a trend toward benefit (p=0.07). Two other uncontrolled trials and one recent preliminary study in MS reported significant therapeutic effects of omega-3 PUFA supplements (see Appendix I). Further studies are needed to determine if omega-3 PUFAs have therapeutic effects in MS. With the available evidence, some MS patients may want to take omega-3 PUFA supplements. If these supplements are taken, it should be emphasized that reasonable doses ($\leq$3 g combined EPA and DHA intake daily) should be taken, vitamin E supplementation may be necessary, this approach should not be used *instead of* disease-modifying medications, and the effects of combination treatment with omega-3 fatty acids and disease-modifying medications in MS have not been well studied.

Additional information:

Dosage: in MS clinical trials, the combined daily intake of EPA and DHA has been 0.9–2.85 g

Contraindications and warnings: bleeding disorders; aspirin sensitivity (decreased pulmonary function); diabetes (high doses may cause hyperglycemia); bipolar disorder and depression (hypomania); pregnancy and lactation (insufficient information)

Major interactions: anticoagulant and antiplatelet medications; oral hypoglycemic medications and insulin (hyperglycemia); antihypertensive medications (hypotension)

Main side effects: generally well tolerated; combined daily intake of EPA and DHA of 3 g or less has been given the "Generally Regarded as Safe" (GRAS) designation by the FDA; fishy taste; belching; halitosis; nosebleeds; bruising; heartburn; high doses may cause nausea and loose stools; since supplementation with PUFAs may produce vitamin E deficiency, supplementation with vitamin E may be necessary (0.6–0.9 IU of vitamin E/g PUFA)

References and additional reading:

Bates D, Cartlidge N, French J, et al. A double-blind controlled trial of long chain n-3 polyunsaturated fatty acids in the treatment of multiple sclerosis. *J Neurol Neurosurg Psych* 1989;52:18–22.

Bowling AC. *Alternative Medicine and Multiple Sclerosis.* New York: Demos Medical Publishing, Inc., 2001:74–90.

Bowling AC, Stewart TM. Current complementary and alternative therapies for multiple sclerosis. *Curr Treat Options Neurol* 2003;5:55–68.

Fragakis AS. *The Health Professional's Guide to Popular Dietary Supplements.* 2nd ed. Chicago, IL: American Dietetic Association, 2003:147–160.

Goldberg P, Fleming M, Picard H. Multiple sclerosis: decreased relapse rate through dietary supplementation with calcium, magnesium and vitamin D. *Med Hyp* 1986;21:193–200.

Jellin JM, Gregory PJ, Batz F, et al. *Pharmacist's Letter/Prescriber's Letter Natural Medicines Comprehensive Database.* 4th ed. Stockton, CA: Therapeutic Research Faculty, 2002:536–541.

Nordvik I, Myhr K-M, Nyland H, et al. Effect of dietary advice and n-3 supplementation in newly diagnosed MS patients. *Acta Neurol Scand* 2000;102:143–149.

Weinstock-Guttman B, Baier M, Peterken L, et al. A randomized study of low-fat diet with w-3 fatty acid supplementation in patients with relapsing-remitting multiple sclerosis (RRMS). *Neurol* 2002;58:A461–2.

FLAXSEED OIL

Other names: flax oil, linseed oil

SUMMARY: Flaxseed oil contains linoleic acid, an omega-6 polyunsaturated fatty acid (PUFA), and alpha-linolenic acid, an omega-3 PUFA. PUFAs, especially omega-3 PUFAs, have mild immunosuppressive effects. Controlled clinical trials indicate that linoleic acid supplements may have mild therapeutic effects in MS (see Appendix I). Studies with omega-3 supplements in MS have been of variable quality; some are suggestive of mild beneficial effects. Further studies are needed to determine if omega-3 and omega-6 PUFAs have therapeutic effects in MS. With the available evidence, some MS patients may choose to take PUFA supplements, such as flaxseed oil. If flaxseed or other PUFA supplements are taken, it should be emphasized that only modest doses should be consumed, vitamin E supplementation may be necessary (0.6–0.9 IU of vitamin E/g PUFA), this approach should not be used *instead of* disease-modifying medications, and combination treatment with PUFAs and disease-modifying medications in MS has not been well studied.

Additional information:

Dosage: 15–30 mL of oil P.O. daily; as a laxative, 1 tablespoon of whole or bruised (not crushed) mature seeds with 6 oz liquid P.O. 2–3 times daily

Contraindications and warnings: bleeding disorders (anticoagulant effect); bowel obstruction (obstruction may be worsened if seeds are consumed without adequate fluid intake); pregnancy and lactation (limited information)

Major interactions: anticoagulant and antiplatelet medications

Main side effects: diarrhea (especially with doses greater than 45 g flaxseed powder daily); flatulence; nausea; excessive doses may produce cyanide toxicity due to immature seedpods that contain cyanogenic nitrates and glucosides, especially linamarin; since supplementation with PUFAs may produce vitamin E deficiency, supplementation with vitamin E may be necessary (0.6–0.9 IU of vitamin E/g PUFA); the safety of long-term use has not been studied

Other considerations: powder and oil are unstable and should be stored in airtight, opaque containers and consumed before the expiration date

References and additional reading:

Bowling AC, Stewart TM. Current complementary and alternative therapies for multiple sclerosis. *Curr Treat Options Neurol* 2003;5:55–68.

Fetrow CW, Avila JR. *Professional's Handbook of Complementary & Alternative Medicines.* 2nd ed. Springhouse, PA: Springhouse Corp, 2001:306–309.

Fragakis AS. *The Health Professional's Guide to Popular Dietary Supplements.* 2nd ed. Chicago, IL: American Dietetic Association, 2003:160–167.

Jellin JM, Gregory PJ, Batz F, et al. *Pharmacist's Letter/Prescriber's Letter Natural Medicines Comprehensive Database.* 4th ed. Stockton, CA: Therapeutic Research Faculty, 2002:541–544.

Peirce A. *Practical Guide to Natural Medicines.* New York: The Stonesong Press, 1999:269–272.

FOLIC ACID

Other names: B complex vitamin, folacin, folate, vitamin B9

SUMMARY: Early studies suggested that folic acid levels may be decreased in serum from MS patients. However, this has not been a consistent finding. Folic acid supplements may decrease the toxicity of methotrexate, which is sometimes used to treat MS. See also Vitamin B12.

Additional information:

Dosage: 1 mg P.O. daily to decrease methotrexate toxicity; RDAs are: adults over 13 years old, 400 mcg; pregnant women, 600 mcg; lactating women, 500 mcg; adults should avoid daily doses greater than 1 mg

Contraindications and warnings: vitamin B12 deficiency (may mask megaloblastic anemia and exacerbate neuropathy); possible worsening of seizure disorders and schizophrenia

Major interactions: may decrease serum levels of phenytoin, fosphenytoin, mysoline, and phenobarbital

Main side effects: generally well tolerated in daily doses of 1 mg or less; high doses may cause altered sleep patterns, vivid dreams, irritability, confusion, worsening of seizures or psychosis, nausea, flatulence, and allergic skin reactions

References and additional reading:

Bowling AC. *Alternative Medicine and Multiple Sclerosis.* New York: Demos Medical Publishing, Inc., 2001:74–194.

Fragakis AS. *The Health Professional's Guide to Popular Dietary Supplements.* 2nd ed. Chicago, IL: American Dietetic Association, 2003:167–175.

Griffith SM, Fisher J, Clarke S, et al. Do patients with rheumatoid arthritis established on methotrexate and folic acid 5 mg daily need to continue folic acid supplements long-term? *Rheumatol* 2000;39:1102–1109.

Isager H. Serum folate in patients with multiple sclerosis. *Acta Neurol Scand* 1970;46:238–242.

Jellin JM, Gregory PJ, Batz F, et al. *Pharmacist's Letter/Prescriber's Letter Natural Medicines Comprehensive Database.* 4th ed. Stockton, CA: Therapeutic Research Faculty, 2002:546–550.

Nijst TQ, Wevers RA, Schoonderwaldt HC, et al. Vitamin B12 and folate concentrations in serum and cerebrospinal fluid of neurological patients with special reference to multiple sclerosis and dementia. *J Neurol Neurosurg Psych* 1990;53:951–954.

Weinblatt ME, Methotrexate. In: Kelley WN, Harris ED, Ruddy S, Sledge CB. *Rheumatology.* Philadelphia: Saunders, 1997:771–786.

GAMMA-LINOLENIC ACID (GLA): see "evening primrose oil"

GARLIC

Other names: ail, ajo, allium, camphor of the poor, clove garlic, nectar of the gods, poor man's treacle, stinking rose

SUMMARY: Garlic may have antihyperlipidemic, antihypertensive, and antifungal properties. However, garlic stimulates T-cells and macrophages; these immune-stimulating effects pose theoretical risks in MS and may interfere with the effects of immune-modulating and immune-suppressing medications. Also, garlic has anticoagulant effects that may interfere with anticoagulant and antiplatelet medications.

References and additional reading:

Bowling AC, Ibrahim R, Stewart TM. Alternative medicine and multiple sclerosis: an objective review from an American perspective. *Int J MS Care* 2000;2:14–21.

Fetrow CW, Avila JR. *Professional's Handbook of Complementary & Alternative Medicines.* 2nd ed. Springhouse, PA: Springhouse Corp, 2001:321–326.

Fragakis AS. *The Health Professional's Guide to Popular Dietary Supplements.* 2nd ed. Chicago, IL: American Dietetic Association, 2003:194–204.

Jellin JM, Gregory PJ, Batz F, et al. *Pharmacist's Letter/Prescriber's Letter Natural Medicines Comprehensive Database.* 4th ed. Stockton, CA: Therapeutic Research Faculty, 2002:571–575.

Lau BH, Yamasake T, Gridley DS. Garlic compounds modulate macrophage and T-lymphocyte functions. *Mol Biother* 1991;3:103–107.

GERMANIUM

Other names: carboxyethylgermanium sesquioxide

SUMMARY: Germanium is sometimes claimed to be an effective therapy for MS. However, it has never been studied in MS and it should be avoided due to multiple possible adverse effects, including renal failure, muscle weakness, peripheral neuropathy, anemia, and death. There have been 31 reports of renal failure or death associated with germanium use.

References and additional reading:

Jellin JM, Gregory PJ, Batz F, et al. *Pharmacist's Letter/Prescriber's Letter Natural Medicines Comprehensive Database.* 4th ed. Stockton, CA: Therapeutic Research Faculty, 2002:583.

GINKGO BILOBA

Other names: adiantifolia, fossil tree, Japanese silver, kew tree, maidenhair tree

SUMMARY: Ginkgo biloba generally refers to ginkgo biloba extract (GBE), an herbal preparation derived from the leaf of the ginkgo tree. GBE is one of the most extensively studied herbal therapies. It contains terpene lactones, which act as antagonists of platelet-activating factor (PAF), and flavonoids, which have antioxidant effects. In patients with probable Alzheimer's disease, GBE may improve cognitive function. PAF has proinflammatory actions. In EAE, one study found that disease severity was worsened by PAF and lessened by GBE. Another study found no effect of PAF antagonists on EAE. Due to the anti-inflammatory effects of GBE, two clinical trials have been conducted to evaluate intravenous ginkgolide B, a terpene lactone component of GBE, as a therapy for MS exacerbations. The initial study, which was small and uncontrolled, reported improvement in attack symptoms in eight out of 10 patients. However, the subsequent study, which was larger (n=104) and controlled, found no therapeutic effect. Therefore, GBE does not appear to be an effective treatment for MS exacerbations. Whether GBE prevents attacks or modifies disease course has not been investigated. Also, there is preliminary evidence that GBE may improve MS-related cognitive dysfunction; further studies are needed in this area.

Additional information:

Dosage: 120–240 mg P.O. daily, divided into two or three doses

Contraindications and warnings: bleeding disorders (anticoagulant effect); possibly seizure disorders (decreased seizure threshold); diabetes; pregnancy and lactation (insufficient information)

Main drug interactions: anticoagulant or antiplatelet medications; thiazide diuretics (hypertension); possibly trazodone (one case report of coma); oral hypoglycemic medications and insulin; may affect cytochrome P450 enzymes (CYP1A2, CYP2D6, and CYP3A4)

Main side effects: gastrointestinal complaints (diarrhea, flatulence, nausea, vomiting); dizziness; headache; rashes; bleeding

References and additional reading:

Bowling AC. *Alternative Medicine and Multiple Sclerosis.* New York: Demos Medical Publishing, Inc., 2001:108–109.

Braquet P, Esanu A, Buisine E, et al. Recent progress in ginkgolide research. *Med Res Rev* 1991;11:295–355.

Brochet B, Guinot P, Orgogozo J, et al. Double-blind, placebo controlled, multi-centre study of ginkgolide B in treatment of acute exacerbations for multiple sclerosis. The Ginkgolide Study Group in multiple sclerosis. *J Neurol Neurosurg Psych* 1995;58:360–362.

Brochet B, Orgogozo J, Guinot P, et al. Étude pilote d'un inhibiteur spécifique du PAF-acéther, le ginkgolide B dans le traitement des poussées aiguës de scléroses en plaques. [Pilot study of ginkgolide B, a PAF-acether specific inhibitor in the treatment of acute outbreaks of multiple sclerosis.] *Rev Neurol (Paris)* 1992;48:229–301.

Ernst E, Pittler MH, Stevinson C, White A. *The Desktop Guide to Complementary and Alternative Medicine: An Evidence-Based Approach*. London: Harcourt Publishers Limited, 2001:114–116.

Fetrow CW, Avila JR. *Professional's Handbook of Complementary & Alternative Medicines*. 2nd ed. Springhouse, PA: Springhouse Corp, 2001:333–337.

Fragakis AS. *The Health Professional's Guide to Popular Dietary Supplements*. 2nd ed. Chicago, IL: American Dietetic Association, 2003:204–211.

Jellin JM, Gregory PJ, Batz F, et al. *Pharmacist's Letter/Prescriber's Letter Natural Medicines Comprehensive Database*. 4th ed. Stockton, CA: Therapeutic Research Faculty, 2002:586–590.

Kenney C, Norman, M, Jacobson M, et al. A double-blind, placebo-controlled, modified crossover pilot study of the effects of ginkgo biloba on cognitive and functional abilities in multiple sclerosis. *Neurol* 2002;58:A458–A459.

Oken B, Storzbach D, Kaye J. The efficacy of ginkgo biloba on cognitive function in Alzheimer disease. *Arch Neurol* 1998;55:1409–1415.

Vela L, Garcia Merino A, Fernandez-Gallardo S, et al. Platelet-activating factor antagonists do not protect against the development of experimental autoimmune encephalomyelitis. *J Neuroimmunol* 1991;33:81–86.

GINSENG: see "Asian ginseng" or "Siberian ginseng"

GLA: see "gamma-linolenic acid" and "evening primrose oil"

GOLDENSEAL

Other names: eye balm, eye root, goldenroot, ground raspberry, hydrastis canadensis, Indian plant, jaundice root, turmeric root, yellow paint, yellow root

SUMMARY: This herb is sometimes claimed to be an effective treatment for viral syndromes and other conditions. It contains berberine, which has sedative properties that could worsen MS fatigue or increase the sedating effects of medications.

References and additional reading:

Bowling AC. *Alternative Medicine and Multiple Sclerosis*. New York: Demos Medical Publishing, Inc., 2001:110.

Fetrow CW, Avila JR. *Professional's Handbook of Complementary & Alternative Medicines*. 2nd ed. Springhouse, PA: Springhouse Corp, 2001:357–360.

Jellin JM, Gregory PJ, Batz F, et al. *Pharmacist's Letter/Prescriber's Letter Natural Medicines Comprehensive Database*. 4th ed. Stockton, CA: Therapeutic Research Faculty, 2002:616–619.

GOTU KOLA

Other names: brahma-buti, centella, gota kola, hydrocotyle, Indian penny-wort, white rot

SUMMARY: This herb, which should not be confused with cola nut (see cola nut), has sedating effects that may worsen MS fatigue or increase the sedating effects of medications.

References and additional reading:

Fetrow CW, Avila JR. *Professional's Handbook of Complementary & Alternative Medicines*. 2nd ed. Springhouse, PA: Springhouse Corp, 2001:364–366.

Jellin JM, Gregory PJ, Batz F, et al. *Pharmacist's Letter/Prescriber's Letter Natural Medicines Comprehensive Database*. 4th ed. Stockton, CA: Therapeutic Research Faculty, 2002:621–623.

GRAPESEED EXTRACT

Other names: activin, extrait de pepins de raisin, leucoanthocyanin, muskat

SUMMARY: Grapeseed extract is sometimes recommended as a therapy for MS. Grapeseed extract, like pinebark extract (pycnogenol), contains oligomeric proanthocyanidins (OPCs), which are antioxidant compounds. At this time, it is unclear whether antioxidants are safe or effective therapies in MS. See also oligomeric proanthocyanidins and pinebark extract.

References and additional reading:

Bowling AC. *Alternative Medicine and Multiple Sclerosis*. New York: Demos Medical Publishing, Inc., 2001:110–111.

Bowling AC, Ibrahim R, Stewart TM. Alternative medicine and multiple sclerosis: an objective review from an American perspective. *Int J MS Care* 2000;2:14–21.

Ernst E, Pittler MH, Stevinson C, White A. *The Desktop Guide to Complementary and Alternative Medicine: An Evidence-Based Approach.* London: Harcourt Publishers Limited, 2001:118–119.

Jellin JM, Gregory PJ, Batz F, et al. *Pharmacist's Letter/Prescriber's Letter Natural Medicines Comprehensive Database.* 4th ed. Stockton, CA: Therapeutic Research Faculty, 2002:627–629.

GREEN TEA

Other names: Chinese tea, matsu-cha

SUMMARY: Green tea contains polyphenols, which have antioxidant effects, and caffeine (10–50 mg caffeine/cup). In modest doses (up to 250 mg daily), caffeine is usually well tolerated and may improve mental alertness. The urinary irritant and diuretic actions of caffeine may worsen MS-associated bladder difficulties. Also, caffeine may be a risk factor for osteoporosis, a condition to which MS patients may be especially prone. For additional information, see caffeine.

References and additional reading:

Fetrow CW, Avila JR. *Professional's Handbook of Complementary & Alternative Medicines.* 2nd ed. Springhouse, PA: Springhouse Corp, 2001:368–371.

Fragakis AS. *The Health Professional's Guide to Popular Dietary Supplements.* 2nd ed. Chicago, IL: American Dietetic Association, 2003:239–246.

Jellin JM, Gregory PJ, Batz F, et al. *Pharmacist's Letter/Prescriber's Letter Natural Medicines Comprehensive Database.* 4th ed. Stockton, CA: Therapeutic Research Faculty, 2002:642–646.

GUARANA

Other names: Brazilian cocoa, paullinia, zoom

SUMMARY: Guarana contains 2.5–7% caffeine, which may increase mental alertness. The effects of guarana and other caffeine-containing products in MS have not been studied. Single doses of guarana contain 200–800 mg; daily intake should not exceed 3 g guarana or approximately 250 mg caffeine. The diuretic and urinary irritant effects of caffeine may provoke MS-related bladder dysfunction. For additional information, see caffeine.

References and additional reading:

Bowling AC. *Alternative Medicine and Multiple Sclerosis.* New York: Demos Medical Publishing, Inc., 2001:103–105.

Jellin JM, Gregory PJ, Batz F, et al. *Pharmacist's Letter/Prescriber's Letter Natural Medicines Comprehensive Database.* 4th ed. Stockton, CA: Therapeutic Research Faculty, 2002:653–656.

HENBANE

Other names: devil's eye, hen bell, hog bean, jupiter's bean, stinking night-shade

SUMMARY: Henbane contains hyoscyamine and scopolamine, which have anticholinergic effects. Use of this herb may increase the anticholinergic effects of anticholinergic medications, including amantadine and tricyclic antidepressants.

References and additional reading:

Jellin JM, Gregory PJ, Batz F, et al. *Pharmacist's Letter/Prescriber's Letter Natural Medicines Comprehensive Database.* 4th ed. Stockton, CA: Therapeutic Research Faculty, 2002:676–678.

HOPS

Other names: common hops, hop strobile

SUMMARY: Hops has sedating properties that may worsen MS fatigue or increase the sedating effects of medications.

References and additional reading:

Fetrow CW, Avila JR. *Professional's Handbook of Complementary & Alternative Medicines.* 2nd ed. Springhouse, PA: Springhouse Corp, 2001:393–397.

Jellin JM, Gregory PJ, Batz F, et al. *Pharmacist's Letter/Prescriber's Letter Natural Medicines Comprehensive Database.* 4th ed. Stockton, CA: Therapeutic research faculty, 2002:689–690.

INOSINE

Other names: hypoxanthine riboside, hypoxanthosine

SUMMARY: Inosine is a precursor of uric acid. Uric acid inhibits reactions mediated by peroxynitrite, a free radical that has been implicated in the pathogenesis of MS and neurodegenerative diseases. In experimental allergic encephalomyelitis (EAE), disease severity is lessened by treatment with uric acid. In a small, uncontrolled study of 11 MS patients, oral inosine increased serum uric acid levels and was associated with clinical improvement in three patients. Further studies in this area are being conducted through a clinical trial at the University of Pennsylvania. Since inosine may cause hyperuricemia, it may aggravate gout, especially with high doses or prolonged use. The long-term effects of inosine are not known.

References and additional reading:

Fetrow CW, Avila JR. *Professional's Handbook of Complementary & Alternative Medicines*. 2nd ed. Springhouse, PA: Springhouse Corp, 2001:415–417.

Jellin JM, Gregory PJ, Batz F, et al. *Pharmacist's Letter/Prescriber's Letter Natural Medicines Comprehensive Database*. 4th ed. Stockton, CA: Therapeutic Research Faculty, 2002:722–723.

Scott GS, Spitsin SV, Kean RB, et al. Therapeutic intervention in experimental allergic encephalomyelitis by administration of uric acid precursors. *Proc Natl Acad Sci* 2002;99:16303–16308.

Spitsin S, Hooper DC, Leist T, et al. Inactivation of peroxynitrite in multiple sclerosis patients after oral administration of inosine may suggest possible approaches to therapy of the disease. *Mult Scler* 2001;7:313–319.

JAMAICAN DOGWOOD

Other names: fishfudle, fish poison bark, West Indian dogwood

SUMMARY: Use of this herb should be avoided because it may be unsafe and there is limited safety information. One of its constituents, rotenone, is a mitochondrial toxin and may be carcinogenic. It has sedative properties that may worsen MS fatigue and increase the sedating effects of medications.

References and additional reading:

Fetrow CW, Avila JR. *Professional's Handbook of Complementary & Alternative Medicines*. 2nd ed. Springhouse, PA: Springhouse Corp, 2001:423–425.

Jellin JM, Gregory PJ, Batz F, et al. *Pharmacist's Letter/Prescriber's Letter Natural Medicines Comprehensive Database*. 4th ed. Stockton, CA: Therapeutic Research Faculty, 2002:740–741.

JIMSON WEED

Other names: angel's trumpet, angel tulip, datura, devil's apple, devil's weed, locoweed, mad apple, moon weed, nightshade, stinkweed, stinkwort, trumpet lily

SUMMARY: Use of this herb should be avoided due to possible anticholinergic toxicity. The anticholinergic effects of the herb may be increased by concomitant use of anticholinergic medications, including amantadine and tricyclic antidepressants.

References and additional reading:

Fetrow CW, Avila JR. *Professional's Handbook of Complementary & Alternative Medicines*. 2nd ed. Springhouse, PA: Springhouse Corp, 2001:428–430.

Jellin JM, Gregory PJ, Batz F, et al. *Pharmacist's Letter/Prescriber's Letter Natural Medicines Comprehensive Database.* 4th ed. Stockton, CA: Therapeutic Research Faculty, 2002:750–752.

KAVA KAVA

Other names: ava, awa, intoxicating pepper, kava pepper, kava root, kawa, kew, tonga, wurzelstock, yagona

SUMMARY: Kava kava is probably effective for the treatment of mild anxiety. It is probably not effective for panic disorder or more severe anxiety disorders. Pharmacologic activity is thought to be due to a class of compounds known as kavalactones or kavapyrones. Kava kava is also sometimes claimed to be effective for insomnia, but its effects on insomnia have only undergone limited investigation. In the past, kava kava was regarded as a generally safe herb. However, in 2001, there were reports of significant liver toxicity. In Germany and Switzerland, the use of kava kava, sometimes on a short-term basis (1–3 months), has been associated with more than 30 cases of liver toxicity, some of which led to liver transplantation or death. Whether these cases were due to kava kava or some contaminant is unclear. Due to these toxic effects, this herb should not be used. If patients take kava kava, they should be warned of possible severe liver toxicity. The risk of liver injury may be potentiated by concomitant administration of hepatotoxic medications, including interferons and methotrexate. Liver function tests should be monitored in patients who choose to take kava kava. Also, this herb has sedating properties that may worsen MS-related fatigue or increase the sedating effects of medications.

Additional information:

Dosage: preparations should be standardized to contain 70% kavalactones; 90–300 mg of kava extract (60–210 mg kavalactones) P.O. daily, divided into three doses

Contraindications and warnings: depression (worsened depression); liver disease (hepatotoxicity); renal disease; neutropenia; thrombocytopenia; pregnancy (decreased uterine tone); lactation (toxic pyrone constituents may pass into breast milk)

Major interactions: alprazolam (coma); sedating medications (excessive sedation); levodopa (decreased levodopa effectiveness)

Main side effects: short-term use of standard dosage may cause severe liver toxicity, sedation, gastrointestinal upset, skin reactions, headaches, and dizziness; very high doses (up to 300–400 g P.O. weekly) may cause ataxia, hair loss, redness of the eyes, respiratory problems, loss of appetite, and difficulties with visual accommodation; prolonged use of high doses may cause kava dermopathy (a pellagra-like disorder characterized by yellowing of the skin, hair, and nails) as well as weight loss, hematuria, decreased platelet and lymphocyte counts, shortness of breath, and possible pulmonary hypertension

References and additional reading:

Bowling AC. *Alternative Medicine and Multiple Sclerosis.* New York: Demos Medical Publishing, Inc., 2001:111.

Ernst E, Pittler MH, Stevinson C, White A. *The Desktop Guide to Complementary and Alternative Medicine: An Evidence-Based Approach.* London: Harcourt Publishers Limited, 2001:128–130.

Fetrow CW, Avila JR. *Professional's Handbook of Complementary & Alternative Medicines.* 2nd ed. Springhouse, PA: Springhouse Corp, 2001:438–441.

Fragakis AS. *The Health Professional's Guide to Popular Dietary Supplements.* 2nd ed. Chicago, IL: American Dietetic Association, 2003:259–264.

Jellin JM, Gregory PJ, Batz F, et al. *Pharmacist's Letter/Prescriber's Letter Natural Medicines Comprehensive Database.* 4th ed. Stockton, CA: Therapeutic Research Faculty, 2002:759–761.

Mischoulon D, Rosenbaum JF. *Natural Medications for Psychiatric Disorders: Considering the Alternatives.* Philadelphia, PA: Lippincott Williams & Wilkins, 2002:128–129.

Russo E. *Handbook of Psychotropic Herbs: A Scientific Analysis of Herbal Remedies for Psychiatric Conditions.* New York: The Haworth Herbal Press, 2001:160–179.

Schulz V, Hänsel R, Tyler VE. *Rational Phytotherapy: A Physicians' Guide to Herbal Medicine.* 3rd ed. Berlin: Springer-Verlag, 1998:65–73.

LEMON BALM

Other names: balm, balm mint, cure-all, dropsy plant, garden balm, honey plant, Melissa, sweet balm, sweet Mary

SUMMARY: This herb has sedating effects that may worsen MS fatigue or increase the sedating effects of medications.

References and additional reading:

Duke JA, Bogenschutz-Godwin MJ, duCellier J, Duke P-AK. *Handbook of Medicinal Herbs.* 2nd ed. Boca Raton, FL: CRC Press, 2002:454–455.

Fetrow CW, Avila JR. *Professional's Handbook of Complementary & Alternative Medicines.* 2nd ed. Springhouse, PA: Springhouse Corp, 2001:459–462.

Jellin JM, Gregory PJ, Batz F, et al. *Pharmacist's Letter/Prescriber's Letter Natural Medicines Comprehensive Database.* 4th ed. Stockton, CA: Therapeutic Research Faculty, 2002:800–802.

LICORICE

Other names: alcacuz, Chinese licorice, gan cao, gan zao, isoflavone, orozuz, regliz, subholz, sweet root

SUMMARY: In the United States, most "licorice" products actually do not contain any licorice (*Glycyrrhiza glabra* species). Instead, they contain anise seed oil, which tastes and smells like licorice and lacks many of the adverse effects of licorice. Other licorice products are "deglycyrrizinated," which means that the active glycyrrhizin constituents have been removed. These products also lack the side effects, and possibly therapeutic effects, of licorice. Chinese herbal medicine (*Glycyrrhiza uralensis* species) and many European licorice products contain authentic licorice. Licorice use may prolong the duration of activity of steroids and may increase the risk of hypokalemia due to steroid use. Licorice has been associated with anti-inflammatory as well as immune-stimulating effects; on a theoretical basis, these actions may worsen or improve MS disease activity and increase or decrease the effectiveness of immune-modulating and immune-suppressing medications. In hepatitis C, glycyrrhizin may increase the effectiveness of interferon-alpha. Use of licorice, especially high doses on a long-term basis, may cause multiple adverse effects, including hypertension, hypokalemia, and pseudoaldosteronism.

References and additional reading:

Duke JA, Bogenschutz-Godwin MJ, duCellier J, Duke P-AK. *Handbook of Medicinal Herbs.* 2nd ed. Boca Raton, FL: CRC Press, 2002:461–464.

Fetrow CW, Avila JR. *Professional's Handbook of Complementary & Alternative Medicines.* 2nd ed. Springhouse, PA: Springhouse Corp, 2001:463–466.

Jellin JM, Gregory PJ, Batz F, et al. *Pharmacist's Letter/ Prescriber's Letter Natural Medicines Comprehensive Database.* 4th ed. Stockton, CA: Therapeutic Research Faculty, 2002:807–810.

Suzuki F, Schmitt DA, Utsunomiya T, et al. Stimulation of host resistance against tumors by glycyrrhizin, an active component of licorice roots. *In Vivo.* 1992;6:589–596.

Yi H, Nakashima I, Isobe K. Enhancement of nitric oxide production from activated macrophages by glycyrrhizin. *Am J Chin Med* 1996;24:271–278.

LOBELIA

Other names: asthma weed, bladderpod, cardinal flower, emetic herb, eye-bright, gagroot, pokeweed, vomit wort, wild tobacco

SUMMARY: This herb is sometimes claimed to be an effective herbal therapy for MS. However, it should be avoided since there is no evidence for its efficacy in MS and it may cause serious adverse effects, including tachycardia, hypotension, seizures, coma, and death.

References and additional reading:

Brinker F. *Herb Contraindications and Drug Interactions.* Sandy, OR: Eclectic Medical Publications, 1998:93–94.

Fetrow CW, Avila JR. *Professional's Handbook of Complementary & Alternative Medicines.* 2nd ed. Springhouse, PA: Springhouse Corp, 2001:469–471.

Jellin JM, Gregory PJ, Batz F, et al. *Pharmacist's Letter/Prescriber's Letter Natural Medicines Comprehensive Database.* 4th ed. Stockton, CA: Therapeutic Research Faculty, 2002:821–822.

MA HUANG: see "ephedra"

MAGNESIUM

Other names: magnesia, Epsom salts

SUMMARY: Magnesium, which is effective for treating constipation and possibly effective for preventing migraine headaches, has been reported to decrease MS-related spasticity. A case report of one MS patient found that oral magnesium glycerophosphate decreased spasticity. Further studies are needed in this area. Interestingly, intravenous magnesium is used to treat tetanus-associated spasms. In reasonable doses, magnesium is usually well tolerated. It may cause gastrointestinal irritation, diarrhea, nausea, and vomiting.

References and additional reading:

Attygale D, Rodrigo N. Magnesium as first line therapy in the management of tetanus: a prospective study of 40 patients. *Anaesthesia* 2002;57;811–817.

Jellin JM, Gregory PJ, Batz F, et al. *Pharmacist's Letter/Prescriber's Letter Natural Medicines Comprehensive Database.* 4th ed. Stockton, CA: Therapeutic Research Faculty, 2002:841–845.

Rossier P, van Erven S, Wade DT. The effect of magnesium oral therapy on spasticity in a patient with multiple sclerosis. *Eur J Neurol* 2000;7:741–744.

MAITAKE MUSHROOM

Other names: dancing mushroom, grifolia, hen of the woods, king of mushrooms, monkey's bench, shelf fungi

SUMMARY: The beta-glucan constituents of maitake mushrooms activate T-cells and produce other immune-stimulating effects that, on a theoretical basis, pose risks in MS and may decrease the effectiveness of immune-modulating and immune-suppressing medications.

References and additional reading:

Jellin JM, Gregory PJ, Batz F, et al. *Pharmacist's Letter/Prescriber's Letter Natural Medicines Comprehensive Database.* 4th ed. Stockton, CA: Therapeutic Research Faculty, 2002:849–850.

Mayell M. Maitake extracts and their therapeutic potential. *Alt Med Rev* 2001;6:48–60.

MANDRAKE

Other names: European mandrake, satan's apple

SUMMARY: This herb, which is sometimes claimed to be an aphrodisiac and to possess magical properties, should be avoided due to possible anticholinergic toxicity. The FDA has banned the sale of mandrake-containing aphrodisiac products. The anticholinergic effects of the herb may be increased by concomitant use of anticholinergic medications, including amantadine and tricyclic antidepressants.

References and additional reading:

Duke JA, Bogenschutz-Godwin MJ, duCellier J, Duke P-AK. *Handbook of Medicinal Herbs.* 2nd ed. Boca Raton, FL: CRC Press, 2002:484–485.

Jellin JM, Gregory PJ, Batz F, et al. *Pharmacist's Letter/Prescriber's Letter Natural Medicines Comprehensive Database.* 4th ed. Stockton, CA: Therapeutic Research Faculty, 2002:513–515.

MARIJUANA

Other names: anashca, banji, cannabis, charas, esrar, ganga, grass, hash, hashish, hemp, kif, pot, sinsemilla, weed

SUMMARY: Marijuana, which is illegal in many states and countries, contains cannabinoids (CBs), pharmacologically active compounds that include tetrahydrocannabinol (THC). Marijuana may be eaten or smoked.

Also, the resin from the plant, which is known as hashish, may be smoked. Orally administered preparations of CBs, available by prescription, include dronabinol (Marinol®), which is THC, in the United States, and nabilone (Cesamet®), a synthetic form of THC, in Canada, Europe, and Australia. CBs have diverse effects. They act on the immune system and nervous system through two receptor systems, CB1 and CB2. CBs also have antioxidant and neuroprotective effects. CBs have immunomodulatory actions and decrease the severity of EAE; the effects of CBs and marijuana on the disease course in MS have not been investigated. Oral CBs and smoked marijuana may improve some MS-related symptoms, including spasticity and pain. In EAE, spasticity and tremor are decreased by CB agonists and increased by CB antagonists. Small clinical studies suggest that smoked marijuana and THC may decrease MS-related spasticity. However, there was no effect of oral CBs on MS-associated spasticity in a controlled trial. Further studies are needed in this area and are being conducted in the United Kingdom. If patients choose to use marijuana, they should be warned of the legal implications and side effects, which include sedation, impaired driving, and, if smoked, cancer and respiratory disease.

Additional information:

Dosage: 1–3 grains (65–195 mg) of marijuana for smoking; 1 grain or less (16–65 mg) of hashish for smoking; in one survey, MS patients smoked marijuana approximately three times daily and six days/week

Contraindications and warnings: cardiovascular disease (cardiac ischemia); respiratory disease (worsened respiratory function); seizure disorders (decreased seizure threshold); immunosuppression (fungal infections due to contamination of marijuana with *Aspergillus* spores); pregnancy (decreased fetal growth, childhood leukemia); lactation (THC is concentrated and excreted in breast milk)

Major interactions: stimulant medications (increased stimulant effect); sedating medications (increased sedating effect); fluoxetine (Prozac®) (hypomania)

Main side effects: nausea and vomiting; sedation; impaired driving for up to eight hours after use; decreased seizure threshold; poor pregnancy outcomes; high doses may cause limb numbness, impair cardiac function, decrease reaction time, and alter visual perception and coordination; chronic use may increase the risk of cancer of the lung, head, and neck, provoke cardiac ischemia, impair pulmonary function, and cause apathy, dependence, bronchitis, and bullous emphysema

References and additional reading:

Achiron A, Miron S, Lavie V, et al. Dexanabinol (HU-211) effect on experimental autoimmune encephalomyelitis: implications for the treatment of acute relapses of multiple sclerosis. *J Neuroimmunol* 2000;102:26–31.

Baker D, Pryce G, Croxford J, et al. Cannabinoids control spasticity and tremor in a multiple sclerosis model. *Nature* 2000;404:84–87.

Bowling AC. *Alternative Medicine and Multiple Sclerosis.* New York: Demos Medical Publishing, Inc., 2001:144–147.

Bowling AC, Ibrahim R, Stewart TM. Alternative medicine and multiple sclerosis an objective review from an American perspective. *Int J MS Care* 2000;2:14–21.

Bowling AC, Stewart TM. Current complementary and alternative therapies for multiple sclerosis. *Curr Treat Options Neurol* 2003;5:55–68.

Consroe P, Musty R, Rein J, et al. The perceived effects of smoked cannabis on patients with multiple sclerosis. *Eur Neurol* 1997;38:44–48.

Francis G. *Marijuana and Medicine.* Totowa, NJ: Humana Press Inc. 1999:631–637.

Hampson AJ, Grimaldi M, Axelrod J, et al. Cannabidiol and (-)delta-9–tetrahydro-cannabinol are neuroprotective antioxidants. *Proc Natl Acad Sci* 1998;95:8268–8273.

Iversen L. *The Science of Marijuana.* New York: Oxford University Press, 2000:155–164.

Jellin JM, Gregory PJ, Batz F, et al. *Pharmacist's Letter/Prescriber's Letter Natural Medicines Comprehensive Database.* 4th ed. Stockton, CA: Therapeutic Research Faculty, 2002:858–860.

Killestein J, Hoogervorst E, Reif M, et al. Safety, tolerability, and efficacy of orally administered cannabinoids in MS. *Neurol* 2002;58:1404–1406.

Parolaro D. Presence and functional regulation of cannabinoid receptors in immune cells. *Life Sci* 1999;65:637–644.

Ungerleider J, Andyrsiak T, Fairbanks L, et al. 9–THC in the treatment of spasticity associated multiple sclerosis. *Adv Alc Subst Abuse* 1987;7:39–50.

Wirguin I, Mechoulam R, Breuer A, et al. Suppression of experimental autoimmune encephalomyelitis by cannabinoid. *Immunopharmacol* 1994;28:209–214.

MATE

Other names: armino, hervea, ilex, Jesuit's Brazil tea, flor de lis, la hoja, la mulata, mate folium, Paraguay tea, St. Bartholemew's tea, union, yerba mate, zerboni

SUMMARY: The leaf and leaf stem of this plant contain 0.2–2% caffeine. Caffeine may increase mental alertness. The effects of mate and other caffeine-containing products have not been investigated in MS. Pyrrolizidine alkaloids, which are hepatotoxic, have been detected in mate. Mate has been associated with hepatotoxicity and increased risk of oropharyngeal and bladder cancer. The hepatotoxic effects may be increased by concomitant use of hepatotoxic medications, including methotrexate and interferons. The diuretic and urinary irritant effects of caffeine may provoke MS-related bladder dysfunction. As a source of caffeine, mate has more risks than caffeine tablets or other caffeine-containing herbs, such as coffee, tea, and guarana. For additional information, see caffeine.

References and additional reading:

Bowling AC. *Alternative Medicine and Multiple Sclerosis*. New York: Demos Medical Publishing, Inc., 2001:103–105.

Fetrow CW, Avila JR. *Professional's Handbook of Complementary & Alternative Medicines*. 2nd ed. Springhouse, PA: Springhouse Corp, 2001:822–825.

Jellin JM, Gregory PJ, Batz F, et al. *Pharmacist's Letter/Prescriber's Letter Natural Medicines Comprehensive Database*. 4th ed. Stockton, CA: Therapeutic Research Faculty, 2002:869–872.

Newall CA, Anderson LA, Phillipson JD. *Herbal Medicines: A Guide for Health-Care Professionals*. London: The Pharmaceutical Press, 1996:189–190.

MEADOWSWEET

Other names: bridewort, dolloff, dropwort, filipendula, gravel root, lady of the meadow, meadow queen, meadow sweet, queen of the meadow, ulmaria

SUMMARY: This herb, which is claimed to be effective for many conditions but does not have documented efficacy for any disease, contains salicylates that may increase the toxicity of methotrexate and may increase the risk of bleeding when taken concomitantly with antiplatelet or anticoagulant medications.

References and additional reading:

Fetrow CW, Avila JR. *Professional's Handbook of Complementary & Alternative Medicines*. 2nd ed. Springhouse, PA: Springhouse Corp, 2001:507–509.

Jellin JM, Gregory PJ, Batz F, et al. *Pharmacist's Letter/Prescriber's Letter Natural Medicines Comprehensive Database*. 4th ed. Stockton, CA: Therapeutic Research Faculty, 2002:872–873.

Newall CA, Anderson LA, Phillipson JD. *Herbal Medicines: A Guide for Health-Care Professionals*. London: The Pharmaceutical Press, 1996:191–192.

MELATONIN

Other names: MEL, pineal hormone, N-acetyl-5–methoxytryptamine

SUMMARY: Melatonin is a hormone produced by the pineal gland. It may be effective for treating jet lag and insomnia. It binds to receptors on T-cells and may activate T-cells. This immune-stimulating effect poses theoretical risks in MS and may interfere with the effects of immune-modulating and immune-suppressing medications. For treating insomnia with dietary supplements, valerian may be safer than melatonin in MS patients.

References and additional reading:

Bowling AC. *Alternative Medicine and Multiple Sclerosis*. New York: Demos Medical Publishing, Inc., 2001:203–204.

Fetrow CW, Avila JR. *Professional's Handbook of Complementary & Alternative Medicines*. 2nd ed. Springhouse, PA: Springhouse Corp, 2001:510–513.

Garcia-Maurino S, Gonzalez-Haba MG, Calvo JR, et al. Melatonin enhances IL-2, IL-6, and IFN-gamma production by human circulating CD4+ cells. *J Immunol* 1997;159:574–581.

Jellin JM, Gregory PJ, Batz F, et al. *Pharmacist's Letter/Prescriber's Letter Natural Medicines Comprehensive Database*. 4th ed. Stockton, CA: Therapeutic Research Faculty, 2002:876–880.

Reiter RJ, Maestroni GJM. Melatonin in relation to the antioxidative defense and immune systems: possible implications for cell and organ transplantation. *J Mol Med* 1999;77:36–39.

MILK THISTLE

Other names: cardui mariae fructus, holy thistle, lady's thistle, silymarin

SUMMARY: This herb, which may decrease liver injury caused by hepato-toxic compounds, has immune-stimulating effects that pose theoretical risks in MS and may decrease the effectiveness of immune-modulating and immune-suppressing medications.

References and additional reading:

Fetrow CW, Avila JR. *Professional's Handbook of Complementary & Alternative Medicines*. 2nd ed. Springhouse, PA: Springhouse Corp, 2001:515–519.

Jellin JM, Gregory PJ, Batz F, et al. *Pharmacist's Letter/Prescriber's Letter Natural Medicines Comprehensive Database*. 4th ed. Stockton, CA: Therapeutic Research Faculty, 2002:889–891.

Wilasrusmee C, Siddiqui J, Bruch D, et al. In vitro immunomodulatory effects of herbal products. *Am Surg* 2002;68:860–864.

MISTLETOE, AMERICAN

Other names: American mistletoe, mistletoe

SUMMARY: Use of this herb should be avoided since it may produce multiple adverse effects, including nausea, bradycardia, hypertension, encephalopathy, and cardiac arrest.

References and additional reading:

Fetrow CW, Avila JR. *Professional's Handbook of Complementary & Alternative Medicines.* 2nd ed. Springhouse, PA: Springhouse Corp, 2001:523–526.

Jellin JM, Gregory PJ, Batz F, et al. *Pharmacist's Letter/Prescriber's Letter Natural Medicines Comprehensive Database.* 4th ed. Stockton, CA: Therapeutic Research Faculty, 2002:63–64.

MISTLETOE, EUROPEAN

Other names: all-heal, birdlime mistletoe, devil's fuge, European mistletoe, helixor, iscador, mistlekraut, vogelmistel

SUMMARY: European mistletoe has been investigated as a cancer therapy and has not been found to be effective. It has immune-stimulating effects that pose theoretical risks in MS and may decrease the effectiveness of immune-modulating and immune-suppressing medications.

References and additional reading:

Fetrow CW, Avila JR. *Professional's Handbook of Complementary & Alternative Medicines.* 2nd ed. Springhouse, PA: Springhouse Corp, 2001:523–526.

Jellin JM, Gregory PJ, Batz F, et al. *Pharmacist's Letter/Prescriber's Letter Natural Medicines Comprehensive Database.* 4th ed. Stockton, CA: Therapeutic Research Faculty, 2002:515–517.

Newall CA, Anderson LA, Phillipson JD. *Herbal Medicines: A Guide for Health-Care Professionals.* London: The Pharmaceutical Press, 1996:193–196.

NIACIN: see "vitamin B3"

NONI JUICE

Other names: Indian mulberry, hog apple, Morinda citrifolia, mulberry, ruibarbo caribe, Tahitian noni juice, bois douleur

SUMMARY: Noni juice is made from the fruit of a Polynesian plant, *Morinda citrifolia.* It is claimed to be an effective treatment for MS, but there are no published clinical trials of its use in MS. It contains polysaccharides that, in limited studies, have been shown to have immune-stimulating effects. These effects pose theoretical risks in MS and may interfere with the effectiveness of immune-modulating and immune-suppressing medications. Since it contains relatively high concentrations of potassium, noni juice may produce hyperkalemia, especially when used in high doses or by patients with renal insufficiency.

References and additional reading:

Fragakis AS. *The Health Professional's Guide to Popular Dietary Supplements*. 2nd ed. Chicago, IL: American Dietetic Association, 2003:308–310.

Hirazumi A, Furusawa E. An immunomodulatory polysaccharide-rich substance from the juice of *Morinda citrifolia* (noni) with antitumour activity. *Phytother Res* 1999;13:380–387.

Jellin JM, Gregory PJ, Batz F, et al. *Pharmacist's Letter/Prescriber's Letter Natural Medicines Comprehensive Database*. 4th ed. Stockton, CA: Therapeutic Research Faculty, 2002:892–894.

Mueller BA, Scott MK, Sowinski KM, et al. Noni juice (Morinda citrifolia): hidden potential for hyperkalemia. *Am J Kidney Dis* 2000;35:310–312.

Solomon N. *Tahitian Noni Juice: How Much, How Often, For What*. Vineyard, UT: Direct Source Publishing, 2000.

OLIGOMERIC PROANTHOCYANIDINS

Other names: OPC

SUMMARY: Oligomeric proanthocyanidins (OPCs), which are constituents in grape seed extract and pinebark extract, are antioxidant compounds that are sometimes recommended as a treatment for MS. However, there are no studies that establish that OPCs or other antioxidants are safe or effective in treating MS. See also grape seed extract and pycnogenol.

References and additional reading:

Bowling AC. *Alternative Medicine and Multiple Sclerosis*. New York: Demos Medical Publishing, Inc., 2001:110–111.

Bowling AC, Ibrahim R, Stewart TM. Alternative medicine and multiple sclerosis: an objective review from an American perspective. *Int J MS Care* 2000;2:14–21.

Ernst E, Pittler MH, Stevinson C, White A. *The Desktop Guide to Complementary and Alternative Medicine: An Evidence-Based Approach*. London: Harcourt Publishers Limited, 2001:118–119.

Jellin JM, Gregory PJ, Batz F, et al. *Pharmacist's Letter/Prescriber's Letter Natural Medicines Comprehensive Database*. 4th ed. Stockton, CA: Therapeutic Research Faculty, 2002:627–629.

OPC: see "oligomeric proanthocyanidins"

PADMA 28

Other names: Badmaev 28, Gabyr-Nirynga

SUMMARY: Padma 28, a complex mixture of more than 20 herbs, is sometimes recommended for treating MS and other diseases. In the late 19th century, two physicians, influenced by Ayurvedic and Tibetan medicine, developed this herbal therapy in Russia. There is limited published information about Padma 28. It appears to have immunosuppressive and antioxidant effects. In one study of mice with EAE, treatment with Padma 28 increased survival times and decreased mortality rates. Only one clinical trial of Padma 28 treatment in MS has been published. In this study, 100 patients with relapsing-remitting and progressive MS were treated for one year with either Padma 28 and symptomatic treatment or with symptomatic treatment only. Clinical improvement was noted in 44% of the treated group and none of the untreated group. Also, deterioration occurred in 12% of the treated group and 40% of the untreated group. There are limitations to this study: an unconventional neurologic grading scale was used; there was not a placebo-treated group; and, important details are not reported, including the criteria used for diagnosing MS and baseline characteristics of patients such as degree of disability and relapse frequency. Further studies are needed to determine the safety and efficacy of Padma 28 in MS.

Additional information:

Dosage: in the only clinical trial reported in MS, two tablets P.O. three times daily

Contraindications and warnings: none known; however, there is limited published information

Major interactions: none known; however, there is limited published information

Main side effects: in the clinical trial in MS, no side effects were reported; no published information on the safety of long-term use

References and additional reading:

Badnaev V, Kozlowski P, Schuller-Levis G, et al. The therapeutic effect of an herbal formula badmaev 28 (padma 28) on experimental allergic encephalomyelitis (EAE) in SJL/J mice. *Phytother Res* 1999;13:218–221.

Bowling AC. *Alternative Medicine and Multiple Sclerosis*. New York: Demos Medical Publishing, Inc., 2001:111–112.

Bowling AC, Stewart TM. Current complementary and alternative therapies for multiple sclerosis. *Curr Treat Options Neurol* 2003;5:55–68.

Korwin-Piotrowska T, Nocon, Stankowska-Chomicz A, et al. Experience of padma 28 in multiple sclerosis. *Phytother Res* 1992;6:133–136.

PASSIONFLOWER

Other names: apricot vine, corona de cristo, fleur de la passion, Jamaican honeysuckle, maypop, passiflora, passion fruit, passion vine, purple passion flower, water lemon, wild passion flower

SUMMARY: This herb has sedating and possibly anxiolytic effects. It is generally well tolerated, but may cause side effects. Its sedating effects may worsen MS fatigue or increase the sedating effects of medications. There are rare reports of vasculitis in association with its use. The leaf of the plant may contain low levels of cyanide.

References and additional reading:

Fetrow CW, Avila JR. *Professional's Handbook of Complementary & Alternative Medicines*. 2nd ed. Springhouse, PA: Springhouse Corp, 2001:580–584.

Jellin JM, Gregory PJ, Batz F, et al. *Pharmacist's Letter/Prescriber's Letter Natural Medicines Comprehensive Database*. 4th ed. Stockton, CA: Therapeutic Research Faculty, 2002:975–977.

PHEASANT'S EYE

Other names: adonis herba, false hellebore, oxeye, red Morocco, sweet vernal

SUMMARY: This herb, which contains cardiac glycosides with digoxin-like activity, is considered poisonous and should not be used. Toxic effects include nausea, vomiting, and cardiac arrhythmias. It may increase the therapeutic and adverse effects of steroids.

References and additional reading:

Duke JA, Bogenschutz-Godwin MJ, duCellier J, Duke P-AK. *Handbook of Medicinal Herbs*. 2nd ed. Boca Raton, FL: CRC Press, 2002:566.

Jellin JM, Gregory PJ, Batz F, et al. *Pharmacist's Letter/Prescriber's Letter Natural Medicines Comprehensive Database*. 4th ed. Stockton, CA: Therapeutic Research Faculty, 2002:997–998.

PINE BARK EXTRACT: see "pycnogenol"

POPLAR

Other names: American aspen, balm of Gilead, populi gemma, quaking aspen

SUMMARY: Poplar is claimed to have anti-inflammatory and multiple other effects, but there is no evidence of efficacy for oral use for any condition. Poplar contains salicylates that may increase the toxicity of methotrexate and may increase the risk of bleeding when taken concomitantly with antiplatelet or anticoagulant medications.

References and additional reading:

Fetrow CW, Avila JR. *Professional's Handbook of Complementary & Alternative Medicines.* 2nd ed. Springhouse, PA: Springhouse Corp, 2001:620–622.

Jellin JM, Gregory PJ, Batz F, et al. *Pharmacist's Letter/Prescriber's Letter Natural Medicines Comprehensive Database.* 4th ed. Stockton, CA: Therapeutic Research Faculty, 2002:1024–1025.

Newall CA, Anderson LA, Phillipson JD. *Herbal Medicines: A Guide for Health-Care Professionals.* London: The Pharmaceutical Press, 1996:218.

PROPOLIS

Other names: bee glue, bee wax, hive dross

SUMMARY: Propolis and other bee products are sometimes recommended for treating MS. Propolis is a waxlike material that is collected by bees from poplar and conifer buds and is used to repair cracks in hives. There are no published studies of its use in MS. It may have weak antiviral and antibacterial activity. Both immune-stimulating and anti-inflammatory effects of propolis have been reported. The immune-stimulating effects pose theoretical risks in MS and may antagonize the effects of immune-suppressing and immune-modulating medications. There is insufficient safety information available.

References and additional reading:

Borrelli F, Maffia P, Pinto L, et al. Phytochemical compounds involved in the anti-inflammatory effect of propolis extract. *Fitoterapia* 2002;73 Suppl 1:S53–S63.

Bowling AC. *Alternative Medicine and Multiple Sclerosis.* New York: Demos Medical Publishing, Inc., 2001:46–51.

Ernst E, Pittler MH, Stevinson C, White A. *The Desktop Guide to Complementary and Alternative Medicine: An Evidence-Based Approach.* London: Harcourt Publishers Limited, 2001:145–147.

Fetrow CW, Avila JR. *Professional's Handbook of Complementary & Alternative Medicines.* 2nd ed. Springhouse, PA: Springhouse Corp, 2001:627–628.

Jellin JM, Gregory PJ, Batz F, et al. *Pharmacist's Letter/Prescriber's Letter Natural Medicines Comprehensive Database.* 4th ed. Stockton, CA: Therapeutic Research Faculty, 2002:1040–1042.

Orsolic N, Basic I. Immunomodulation by water-soluble derivative of propolis: a factor of antitumor activity. *J Ethnopharmacol* 2003;84:265–273.

Peirce A. *Practical Guide to Natural Medicines.* New York: The Stonesong Press, 1999:518–520.

PSYLLIUM

Other names: black plantago, black psyllium, blond plantago, blond psyllium, Englishman's foot, fleaseed, fleawort, ispaghula, ispagol, plantago, plantain

SUMMARY: Psyllium, which is derived from the seeds of black psyllium (*Plantago psyllium*) and blond psyllium (*Plantago ovata*), has been FDA approved as a laxative. It is generally safe, but it may cause esophageal or intestinal obstruction if fluid intake is inadequate. MS patients who are prone to constipation may consider using it. Psyllium also lowers serum cholesterol levels. Psyllium must be taken with adequate fluid, should not be used by patients with dysphagia, and may alter levels of carbamazepine (Tegretol®) and other medications.

Additional information:

Dosage: variable dosage; start with small amounts and increase to desired response; as a laxative, 10–30 g of seeds P.O. daily, in divided doses; to avoid esophageal and intestinal obstruction, should be taken with at least 150 mL water for each 5 g of seed; the FDA recommends at least 8 oz of water or other liquid with each dose; should be taken one hour after consuming a meal or taking medications; seeds should not be crushed since this may release a nephrotoxic pigment (this pigment has been removed from most commercial products); non-commercial products should not be used because they may contain nephrotoxic compounds

Contraindications and warnings: diabetes (hypoglycemia); dysphagia (choking); intestinal obstruction; renal disease (nephrotoxicity)

Major interactions: insulin and oral hypoglycemic medications (hypoglycemia); decreased absorption of carbamazepine (Tegretol®), digoxin, lithium, warfarin (Coumadin®), and possibly other drugs; to avoid decreased or delayed absorption, oral medications should be taken one hour before or four hours after psyllium

Main side effects: if fluid intake is inadequate, choking and intestinal obstruction are possible; flatulence; abdominal distention; possible nephrotoxicity if seeds are crushed; the FDA requires that psyllium products have this precaution: "WARNING: Taking this product without adequate fluid may cause it to swell and block your throat or esophagus and may cause choking. Do not take this product if you have difficulty in swallowing. If you experience chest pain, choking, vomiting, or difficulty in swallowing or breathing after taking this product, seek immediate medical attention."

References and additional reading:

Bowling AC. *Alternative Medicine and Multiple Sclerosis.* New York: Demos Medical Publishing, Inc., 2001:112–113.

Brinker F. *Herb Contraindications and Drug Interactions.* Sandy, OR: Eclectic Medical Publications, 1998:114.

Fetrow CW, Avila JR. *Professional's Handbook of Complementary & Alternative Medicines.* 2nd ed. Springhouse, PA: Springhouse Corp, 2001:610–615.

Jellin JM, Gregory PJ, Batz F, et al. *Pharmacist's Letter/Prescriber's Letter Natural Medicines Comprehensive Database.* 4th ed. Stockton, CA: Therapeutic Research Faculty, 2002:175–177, 192–194.

Peirce A. *Practical Guide to Natural Medicines.* New York: The Stonesong Press, 1999:520–523.

PYCNOGENOL

Other names: condensed tannins, French maritime pine bark extract, leucoanthocyanidins, oligomeric proanthocyanidins, OPC, OPCs, PCO, PCOs, pine bark extract, procyandiol oligomers, procyandolic oligomers, pygenol

SUMMARY: Pycnogenol is a registered trademark in the United States for an extract derived from French maritime pine bark (*Pinus maritima*). Pycnogenol is sometimes claimed to be an effective MS therapy. However, there are no clinical studies of pycnogenol use in MS. Also, pycnogenol, like grape seed extract, contains flavonoid compounds known as oligomeric proanthocyanidins (OPCs), which have antioxidant effects. There are no studies that demonstrate that pycnogenol, OPCs, or other antioxidants are safe or effective in treating MS. See also grapeseed extract and oligomeric proanthocyanidins.

References and additional reading:

Bowling AC. *Alternative Medicine and Multiple Sclerosis*. New York: Demos Medical Publishing, Inc., 2001:113.

Fetrow CW, Avila JR. *Professional's Handbook of Complementary & Alternative Medicines*. 2nd ed. Springhouse, PA: Springhouse Corp, 2001:607–608.

Jellin JM, Gregory PJ, Batz F, et al. *Pharmacist's Letter/Prescriber's Letter Natural Medicines Comprehensive Database*. 4th ed. Stockton, CA: Therapeutic Research Faculty, 2002:1047–1049.

Peirce A. *Practical Guide to Natural Medicines*. New York: The Stonesong Press, 1999:525–527.

PYRIDOXINE: see "vitamin B6"

REISHI MUSHROOM

Other names: holy mushroom, ling chih, ling zhi cao, mannentake, mushroom of immortality, mushroom of spiritual potency, rei-shi, spirit plant

SUMMARY: This mushroom, known as "the elixir of life," includes two species, *Ganoderma lucidum* and *Ganoderma japonicum*. It is a component of some traditional Chinese herbal therapies. It has immune-stimulating effects that may pose theoretical risks in MS and may interfere with the effectiveness of immune-modulating and immune-suppressing medications.

References and additional reading:

Duke JA, Bogenschutz-Godwin MJ, duCellier J, Duke P-AK. *Handbook of Medicinal Herbs*. 2nd ed. Boca Raton, FL: CRC Press, 2002:620.

Jellin JM, Gregory PJ, Batz F, et al. *Pharmacist's Letter/Prescriber's Letter Natural Medicines Comprehensive Database*. 4th ed. Stockton, CA: Therapeutic Research Faculty, 2002:1075–1076.

Peirce A. *Practical Guide to Natural Medicines*. New York: The Stonesong Press, 1999:542–544.

Wang SY, Hsu HL, Hsu HC, et al. The anti-tumor effect of *Ganoderma lucidum* is mediated by cytokines released from activated macrophages and T lymphocytes. *Int J Cancer* 1997;70:699–705.

RIBOFLAVIN: see "vitamin B2"

ROYAL JELLY

Other names: bee saliva, bee spit, honey bee milk, queen bee jelly

SUMMARY: Royal jelly is sometimes claimed to be an effective therapy for MS. It is a milky secretion that is produced by pharyngeal glands of young honey bees and is used to nurture queen bees. There is no evidence to support its use in MS. It is usually well tolerated. However, in individuals with asthma or allergies, it may cause allergic symptoms, including pruritis, urticaria, eczema, conjunctivitis, rhinorrhea, dyspnea, facial and eyelid edema, and asthma. Rarely, it may cause more severe side effects such as status asthmaticus, anaphylaxis, and death.

References and additional reading:

Bowling AC. *Alternative Medicine and Multiple Sclerosis*. New York: Demos Medical Publishing, Inc., 2001:46–51.

Fetrow CW, Avila JR. *Professional's Handbook of Complementary & Alternative Medicines*. 2nd ed. Springhouse, PA: Springhouse Corp, 2001:668–670.

Fragakis AS. *The Health Professional's Guide to Popular Dietary Supplements*. 2nd ed. Chicago, IL: American Dietetic Association, 2003: 332–335.

Jellin JM, Gregory PJ, Batz F, et al. *Pharmacist's Letter/Prescriber's Letter Natural Medicines Comprehensive Database*. 4th ed. Stockton, CA: Therapeutic Research Faculty, 2002:1097–1098.

S-ADENOSYLMETHIONINE: see "SAMe"

SAFFLOWER SEED OIL

Other names: American saffron, azafran, bastard saffron, benibana, dyer's saffron, fake saffron, hing hua, zaffer, zafran

SUMMARY: Safflower seed oil, like sunflower seed oil, contains relatively high concentrations (75%) of linoleic acid, an omega-six polyunsaturated fatty acid (PUFA). Other constituents include oleic acid (13%), palmitic acid (6%), stearic acid (3%), and a mixture of saturated fatty acids. Controlled clinical trials indicate that linoleic acid (LA) supplementation may mildly decrease relapse severity and disease progression in relapsing-remitting MS (see Appendix I). Most of the LA supplementation trials have used sunflower seed oil; presumably, safflower seed oil would have similar effects. It has been argued that gamma-linolenic acid (GLA), another omega-6 PUFA found in evening primrose oil, borage seed oil, and black currant seed oil, may be a more physiologically useful PUFA than LA. If PUFA supplements are consumed on a regular basis, vitamin E supplements (0.6–0.9 IU of vitamin E/g PUFA) should be taken to prevent vitamin E deficiency.

Additional information:

Dosage: in studies of relapsing-remitting MS, daily doses of 17–23 g of sunflower seed oil P.O. were used

Contraindications and warnings: bleeding disorders (increased risk of bleeding)

Major interactions: antiplatelet and anticoagulant medications (increased risk of bleeding)

Main side effects: usually well tolerated; the safety of long-term use of high doses is not known; since supplementation with PUFAs may produce vitamin E deficiency, supplementation with vitamin E may be necessary (0.6–0.9 IU of vitamin E/g PUFA)

References and additional reading:

Bates D, Fawcett P, Shaw D, et al. Polyunsaturated fatty acids in treatment of acute remitting multiple sclerosis. *Br Med J* 1978;2:1390–1391.

Bates D, Fawcett P, Shaw D, et al. Trial of polyunsaturated fatty acids in non-relapsing multiple sclerosis. *Br Med J* 1977;2:932–933.

Bowling AC. *Alternative Medicine and Multiple Sclerosis*. New York: Demos Medical Publishing, Inc., 2001:74–90.

Bowling AC, Stewart TM. Current complementary and alternative therapies for multiple sclerosis. *Curr Treat Options Neurol* 2003;5:55–68.

Dworkin R, Bates D, Millar J, et al. Linoleic acid and multiple sclerosis: a reanalysis of three double-blind trials. Neurol 1984;34:1441–1445.

Fetrow CW, Avila JR. *Professional's Handbook of Complementary & Alternative Medicines*. 2nd ed. Springhouse, PA: Springhouse Corp, 2001:673–675.

Jellin JM, Gregory PJ, Batz F, et al. *Pharmacist's Letter/Prescriber's Letter Natural Medicines Comprehensive Database*. 4th ed. Stockton, CA: Therapeutic Research Faculty, 2002:1105–1106.

Millar J, Zilkha K, Langman M, et al. Double-blind trial of linoleate supplementation of the diet in multiple sclerosis. *Br Med J* 1973;1:765–768.

Paty D. Double-blind trial of linoleic acid in multiple sclerosis. *Arch Neurol* 1983;40:693–694.

SAGE

Other names: common sage, dalmatian sage, garden sage, meadow sage, sauge, scarlet sage, Spanish sage, tree sage, true sage

SUMMARY: Sage is used for a variety of conditions, especially gastrointestinal. It has sedative properties that may worsen MS fatigue or increase the sedating effects of medications. Also, sage may increase the risk of seizures and have mild hypoglycemic effects.

References and additional reading:

Fetrow CW, Avila JR. *Professional's Handbook of Complementary & Alternative Medicines.* 2nd ed. Springhouse, PA: Springhouse Corp, 2001:677–679.

Jellin JM, Gregory PJ, Batz F, et al. *Pharmacist's Letter/Prescriber's Letter Natural Medicines Comprehensive Database.* 4th ed. Stockton, CA: Therapeutic Research Faculty, 2002:1108–1109.

Newall CA, Anderson LA, Phillipson JD. *Herbal Medicines: A Guide for Health-Care Professionals.* London: The Pharmaceutical Press, 1996:231–232.

ST. JOHN'S WORT

Other names: amber, demon chaser, devil's scourge, goatweed, God's wonder plant, grace of God, hardhay, *Hypericum*, klamath weed, rosin rose, SJW, tipton weed, witches' herb

SUMMARY: St. John's wort (SJW) may be effective for treating mild to moderate depression, a condition that occurs frequently in MS. Interestingly, in one study, SJW decreased release of interleukin-6 (IL-6), a cytokine that probably mediates the flu-like side effects of beta-interferons. SJW has sedating properties that may worsen MS fatigue or increase the sedating effects of medications. Photosensitivity may occur, especially in fair-skinned individuals. Since SJW induces cytochrome P450 (CYP3A4, CYP2D6, CYP1A2) and intestinal P-glycoprotein/multi-drug resistance (MDR-1) drug transporter, interactions are possible with many drugs, including antidepressant medications, anticonvulsants, and oral contraceptives (see "Additional Information"). SJW should not be taken with other antidepressant medications. Patients should not diagnose and treat their own depression.

Additional information:

Dosage: 300 mg P.O. three times daily in most clinical trials for depression; for unclear reasons, labels on SJW bottles may recommend lower dosages; extracts should be standardized to contain 0.3% hypericin

Contraindications and warnings: bipolar disorder (mania or hypomania); depression (hypomania); Alzheimer's disease (psychosis); schizophrenia (psychosis); possibly infertility (inhibition of oocyte fertilization and altered sperm DNA); pregnancy (decreased uterine tone); lactation (colic and lethargy in nursing infants)

Major interactions: antidepressant medications, including tricyclic antidepressants, SSRIs, trazodone, nefazodone (Serzone®), and MAO inhibitors; serotonergic medications, including 5HT1 agonists (triptans), fenfluramine (Pondimin®), SSRIs, trazodone, and nefazodone (Serzone®); sedating medications, including benzodiazepines, lioresal (Baclofen®), tizanidine (Zanaflex®), narcotics, and barbiturates; photosensitizing drugs, including amitriptyline, quinolones, sulfa drugs, and tetracycline; calcium channel blockers; cyclosporin (Neoral®, Sandimmune®); digoxin; protease inhibitors; oral contraceptives; theophylline; warfarin (Coumadin®)

Main side effects: generally well tolerated; fatigue; insomnia; vivid dreams; restlessness; anxiety; irritability; gastrointestinal discomfort; dry mouth; headache; dizziness; paresthesias; abrupt discontinuation may produce withdrawal effects, including headache, nausea, dizziness, insomnia, paresthesias, confusion, and fatigue

References and additional reading:

Bowling AC. *Alternative Medicine and Multiple Sclerosis*. New York: Demos Medical Publishing, Inc., 2001:113–115.

Bowling AC, Ibrahim R, Stewart TM. Alternative medicine and multiple sclerosis: an objective review from an American perspective. *Int J MS Care* 2000;2:14–21.

Fetrow CW, Avila JR. *Professional's Handbook of Complementary & Alternative Medicines*. 2nd ed. Springhouse, PA: Springhouse Corp, 2001:746–750.

Fragakis AS. *The Health Professional's Guide to Popular Dietary Supplements*. 2nd ed. Chicago, IL: American Dietetic Association, 2003:334–350.

Jellin JM, Gregory PJ, Batz F, et al. *Pharmacist's Letter/Prescriber's Letter Natural Medicines Comprehensive Database*. 4th ed. Stockton, CA: Therapeutic Research Faculty, 2002:1180–1184.

Mischoulon D, Rosenbaum JF. *Natural Medications for Psychiatric Disorders: Considering the Alternatives*. Philadelphia, PA: Lippincott Williams & Wilkins, 2002:3–12.

Russo E. *Handbook of Psychotropic Herbs: A Scientific Analysis of Herbal Remedies for Psychiatric Conditions*. New York: The Haworth Herbal Press, 2001:55–73.

Thiele B, Brink I, Ploch M. Modulation of cytokine expression by hypericum extract. *J Geriatr Psych Neurol* 1994;7(suppl 1):S60–S62.

SAMe

Other names: ademetionine, adenosylmethionine, S-adenosylmethionine, sammy

SUMMARY: SAMe, which functions as a methyl group donor for a wide range of compounds, is possibly effective in the treatment of depression and the symptoms of osteoarthritis and fibromyalgia. On theoretical grounds, it has been claimed that it may be an effective treatment for MS and several other neurologic diseases. There are no published clinical trials of SAMe use in MS. SAMe should not be taken with antidepressant medications. SAMe is involved in homocysteine metabolism; at this time it is unclear whether SAMe supplementation increases or decreases serum homocysteine levels. Patients should not diagnose and treat their own depression.

Additional information:

Dosage: 400–1600 mg P.O. daily for depression

Contraindications and warnings: bipolar disease (mania or hypomania); hyperhomocysteinemia; pregnancy and lactation (insufficient information)

Major interactions: antidepressant medications, including SSRIs, tricyclics, and MAO inhibitors; steroids (increased adverse and therapeutic effects)

Main side effects: generally well tolerated; no serious toxicity reported in 22,000 patients taking SAMe; flatulence; nausea; vomiting; diarrhea; headache; anxiety; hypomania; possibly hyperhomocysteinemia

References and additional reading:

Bowling AC. *Alternative Medicine and Multiple Sclerosis.* New York: Demos Medical Publishing, Inc., 2001:204–205.

Bottiglieri T, Hyland K, Reynolds EH. The clinical potential of ademetionine (S-adenosylmethionine) in neurological disorders. *Drugs* 1994;48:137–152.

Fetrow CW, Avila JR. *Professional's Handbook of Complementary & Alternative Medicines.* 2nd ed. Springhouse, PA: Springhouse Corp, 2001:679–688.

Jellin JM, Gregory PJ, Batz F, et al. *Pharmacist's Letter/Prescriber's Letter Natural Medicines Comprehensive Database.* 4th ed. Stockton, CA: Therapeutic Research Faculty, 2002:1110–1113.

Mischoulon D, Rosenbaum JF. *Natural Medications for Psychiatric Disorders: Considering the Alternatives.* Philadelphia, PA: Lippincott Williams & Wilkins, 2002:3–51.

SASSAFRAS

Other names: ague tree, cinnamon wood, kuntze saloop, lignum floridum, root bark, saxifrax

SUMMARY: This herb, which was used in the past to flavor root beer, is claimed to be effective for inflammation, infections, urinary tract disorders, and several other conditions. There is no evidence that it is effective for any

condition. It may actually act as a urinary tract irritant. Also, it has sedative properties that may worsen MS-related fatigue or increase the sedative
effects of medications. Safrole, a component of sassafras, is a hepatic car-
cinogen and cytochrome P450 inducer; safrole-free extracts are available,
but these are also carcinogenic in animal models. The use of this herb
should be avoided.

References and additional reading:

Fetrow CW, Avila JR. *Professional's Handbook of Complementary & Alternative
    Medicines.* 2nd ed. Springhouse, PA: Springhouse Corp, 2001:692–694.

Jellin JM, Gregory PJ, Batz F, et al. *Pharmacist's Letter/Prescriber's Letter Natural
    Medicines Comprehensive Database.* 4th ed. Stockton, CA: Therapeutic
    Research Faculty, 2002:1119–1120.

Newall CA, Anderson LA, Phillipson JD. *Herbal Medicines: A Guide for Health-Care
    Professionals.* London: The Pharmaceutical Press, 1996:235–236.

Peirce A. *Practical Guide to Natural Medicines.* New York: The Stonesong Press,
    1999:575–577.

SAW PALMETTO

Other names: American dwarf palm tree, cabbage palm, sabal fructus

SUMMARY: Saw palmetto, a component of the herbal combination product known as "PC-SPES," is probably an effective treatment for symptoms
of benign prostatic hypertrophy (BPH). The active constituent, the lipo-
sterolic extract of *Serenoa repens* (LSESR), inhibits 5–alpha-reductase in a
manner similar to that of finasteride (Proscar®), the prescription medica-
tion for BPH. If used for BPH, it should be used under the guidance of a
healthcare professional. There is very limited *in vitro* evidence that polysaccharides in saw palmetto have immune-stimulating effects; in theory,
these effects pose risks in MS and may decrease the effectiveness of
immune-modulating and immune-suppressing medications.

References and additional reading:

Fetrow CW, Avila JR. *Professional's Handbook of Complementary & Alternative
    Medicines.* 2nd ed. Springhouse, PA: Springhouse Corp, 2001:696–699.

Jellin JM, Gregory PJ, Batz F, et al. *Pharmacist's Letter/Prescriber's Letter Natural
    Medicines Comprehensive Database.* 4th ed. Stockton, CA: Therapeutic
    Research Faculty, 2002:1121–1123.

Newall CA, Anderson LA, Phillipson JD. *Herbal Medicines: A Guide for Health-Care
    Professionals.* London: The Pharmaceutical Press, 1996:237–238.

Peirce A. *Practical Guide to Natural Medicines.* New York: The Stonesong Press,
    1999:579–581.

Wagner H, Flachsbarth H. A new antipholigistic principle from *Saba serrulata*, I. *Planta Medica*. 1981;41:244–251.

SCOPOLIA

Other names: belladonna

SUMMARY: Use of this herb should be avoided due to possible anticholinergic toxicity. The anticholinergic effects of the herb may be increased by concomitant use of anticholinergic medications, including amantadine and tricyclic antidepressants.

References and additional reading:

Duke JA, Bogenschutz-Godwin MJ, duCellier J, Duke P-AK. *Handbook of Medicinal Herbs*. 2nd ed. Boca Raton, FL: CRC Press, 2002:657.

Jellin JM, Gregory PJ, Batz F, et al. *Pharmacist's Letter/Prescriber's Letter Natural Medicines Comprehensive Database*. 4th ed. Stockton, CA: Therapeutic Research Faculty, 2002:1126–1127.

SCULLCAP

Other names: blue pimpernel, helmet flower, hoodwort, mad weed, maddog weed, quaker bonnet, scutelluria

SUMMARY: This herb is sometimes claimed to be an effective treatment for MS. It is also sometimes recommended for spasticity, stroke, movement disorders, seizures, and several other conditions. Currently, there are no studies supporting its use in MS or any other condition. There are preliminary promising results in stroke. There are several reports of severe hepatotoxicity associated with the use of scullcap-containing products; it is not clear if these were due to scullcap or to hepatotoxic adulterants such as germander (*Teucrium* species). One case of fatal hepatotoxicity involved a 28–year-old man with mild MS who took scullcap, another herb (pau d'arco), and zinc. The hepatotoxic effects of scullcap may be increased by hepatotoxic medications, including methotrexate and interferons. Scullcap has sedating properties that may worsen MS fatigue or increase the sedating effects of medications.

References and additional reading:

Duke JA, Bogenschutz-Godwin MJ, duCellier J, Duke P-AK. *Handbook of Medicinal Herbs*. 2nd ed. Boca Raton, FL: CRC Press, 2002:673.

Fetrow CW, Avila JR. *Professional's Handbook of Complementary & Alternative Medicines*. 2nd ed. Springhouse, PA: Springhouse Corp, 2001:703–706.

Hullar TE, Sapers BL, Ridker PM, et al. Herbal toxicity and fatal hepatic failure. *Am J Med* 1999;106:267–268.

Jellin JM, Gregory PJ, Batz F, et al. *Pharmacist's Letter/Prescriber's Letter Natural Medicines Comprehensive Database.* 4th ed. Stockton, CA: Therapeutic Research Faculty, 2002:1132–1333.

SELENIUM

Other names: selenite, selenium dioxide

SUMMARY: Selenium has antioxidant effects and may prevent certain forms of cancer. Like many other antioxidants, it has immune-stimulating effects that pose theoretical risks in MS and may decrease the effectiveness of immune-modulating and immune-suppressing medications. In one EAE study, high selenium intake worsened disease severity and increased mortality rate relative to normal selenium intake. Selenium deficiency had no effect on EAE severity. A five-week study of 18 people with MS reported no adverse effects with supplementation with selenium, vitamin C, and vitamin E. Further studies are needed to evaluate the possible effects of selenium and other antioxidants in MS. If selenium is taken by MS patients, it may be best to use modest doses (50 mcg or less daily). Doses greater than 400 mcg daily should be avoided.

Additional information:

Dosage: 200 mcg P.O. daily for cancer prevention; the RDAs are: adults, 55 mcg; pregnant women, 60 mcg; lactating women, 70 mcg; the Tolerable Upper Intake Level (UL) is 400 mcg P.O. daily

Contraindications and warnings: immune-stimulating effect may pose theoretical risks in MS and other diseases associated with increased immune system activity; avoid high doses (> 60 mcg) during pregnancy (possible teratogenic effects and spontaneous abortion); avoid high doses (> 70 mcg) during lactation

Major interactions: cisplatin (Platinol-AQ®) (increased cytotoxic effect); in theory, possible decreased effectiveness of immune-modulating and immune-suppressing medications

Main side effects: generally well tolerated in reasonable doses; possible side effects include fatigue, nausea, vomiting, nail changes, and irritability; high doses may cause symptoms similar to arsenic toxicity, including hair loss, white horizontal streaking on fingernails, fatigue, irritability, paronychia, nausea, vomiting, hyperreflexia, and metallic taste; other symptoms of selenium poisoning are tremor, muscle tenderness, facial flushing, thrombocytopenia, and hepatorenal dysfunction

References and additional reading:

Bowling AC. *Alternative Medicine and Multiple Sclerosis.* New York: Demos Medical Publishing, Inc., 2001:187–189, 196.

Bowling AC, Ibrahim R, Stewart TM. Alternative medicine and multiple sclerosis: an objective review from an American perspective. *Int J MS Care* 2000;2:14–21.

Bowling AC, Stewart TM. Current complementary and alternative therapies for multiple sclerosis. *Curr Treat Options Neurol* 2003;5:55–68.

Fragakis AS. *The Health Professional's Guide to Popular Dietary Supplements.* 2nd ed. Chicago, IL: American Dietetic Association, 2003:353–359.

Jellin JM, Gregory PJ, Batz F, et al. *Pharmacist's Letter/Prescriber's Letter Natural Medicines Comprehensive Database.* 4th ed. Stockton, CA: Therapeutic Research Faculty, 2002:1137–1138.

Kiremidjian-Schumacher L, Roy M, Wishe HI, et al. Regulation of cellular immune responses by selenium. *Biol Trace Elem Res* 1992;33:23–35.

Mai J, Sorenson P, Hansen J. High dose antioxidant supplementation to MS patients: effects on glutathione peroxidase, clinical safety, and absorption of selenium. *Biol Trace Elem Res* 1990;24:109–117.

Peirce A. *Practical Guide to Natural Medicines.* New York: The Stonesong Press, 1999:586–588.

Scelsi R, Savoldi F, Ceroni M, et al. Selenium and experimental allergic encephalomyelitis. *J Neurol Scis* 1983;61:369–379.

SENEGA

Other names: Chinese senega, mountain flax, milkwort, mountain polygala, rattlesnake root, seneca, snake root

SUMMARY: Seneca Indians and other North American tribes chewed senega root and then applied the pulp to rattlesnake bites. Senega is claimed to be an effective treatment for MS and several other conditions. There is a French patent that claims that a triterpenic acid extract from senega has anti-inflammatory activity and is effective in treating MS, psoriasis, eczema, and graft rejection. There are not any published studies to support its use in MS. Senega may cause nausea, vomiting, and diarrhea.

References and additional reading:

Fetrow CW, Avila JR. *Professional's Handbook of Complementary & Alternative Medicines.* 2nd ed. Springhouse, PA: Springhouse Corp, 2001:710–713.

Jellin JM, Gregory PJ, Batz F, et al. *Pharmacist's Letter/Prescriber's Letter Natural Medicines Comprehensive Database.* 4th ed. Stockton, CA: Therapeutic Research Faculty, 2002:1140–1141.

Newall CA, Anderson LA, Phillipson JD. *Herbal Medicines: A Guide for Health-Care Professionals*. London: The Pharmaceutical Press, 1996:241–242.

Peirce A. *Practical Guide to Natural Medicines*. New York: The Stonesong Press, 1999:588–590.

SENNA

Other names: Alexandrian senna, casse, Cassia senna, Indian senna

SUMMARY: Senna, obtained from the leaf and root of the *Senna alexandrina* plant, acts as a stimulant laxative, and is effective for treating constipation. It may produce potassium depletion and increase the hypokalemic effects of steroids. Long-term use (more than one to two weeks) should be avoided because it may cause "laxative-dependency syndrome" and increase the risk of colorectal cancer and other cancer types.

Additional information:

Dosage: for short-term use (less than one to two weeks) only; two tablets (187 mg) P.O. at bedtime; one cup of tea (0.5–2 g of herb/cup of water) once or twice daily

Contraindications and warnings: hypokalemia; gastrointestinal inflammatory conditions; hemorrhoids; anal prolapse; dehydration; pregnancy and lactation

Major interactions: cardiac glycosides (due to hypokalemia); oral medications generally (possibly decreased absorption)

Main side effects: discolored urine; long-term use (more than one to two weeks) may cause "laxative-dependency syndrome" (decreased gastric motility, nonfunctioning colon, laxative-induced diarrhea) and possibly increase the risk of colorectal cancer and other forms of cancer

References and additional reading:

Brinker F. Herb *Contraindications and Drug Interactions*. Sandy, OR: Eclectic Medical Publications, 1998:121–122.

Fetrow CW, Avila JR. *Professional's Handbook of Complementary & Alternative Medicines*. 2nd ed. Springhouse, PA: Springhouse Corp, 2001:713–716.

Jellin JM, Gregory PJ, Batz F, et al. *Pharmacist's Letter/Prescriber's Letter Natural Medicines Comprehensive Database*. 4th ed. Stockton, CA: Therapeutic Research Faculty, 2002:1141–1142.

Newall CA, Anderson LA, Phillipson JD. *Herbal Medicines: A Guide for Health-Care Professionals*. London: The Pharmaceutical Press, 1996:243–244.

Peirce A. *Practical Guide to Natural Medicines*. New York: The Stonesong Press, 1999:590–592.

SHEPHERD'S PURSE

Other names: blind weed, capsella, caseweed, cocowort, lady's purse, mother's heart, pepper-and-salt, pick-pocket, rattle pouches, sanguinary, shepherd's sprout, shovelweed, St. James' weed, toywort, witches' pouches

SUMMARY: This herb, claimed to be effective for cardiac conditions, painful menstruation, bleeding, and other conditions, has not been proven to be effective for any condition. It has multiple possible side effects, including sedating properties that may worsen MS fatigue and increase the sedating effects of medications.

References and additional reading:

Fetrow CW, Avila JR. *Professional's Handbook of Complementary & Alternative Medicines.* 2nd ed. Springhouse, PA: Springhouse Corp, 2001:720–722.

Jellin JM, Gregory PJ, Batz F, et al. *Pharmacist's Letter/Prescriber's Letter Natural Medicines Comprehensive Database.* 4th ed. Stockton, CA: Therapeutic Research Faculty, 2002:1146–1147.

Newall CA, Anderson LA, Phillipson JD. *Herbal Medicines: A Guide for Health-Care Professionals.* London: The Pharmaceutical Press, 1996:245–246.

SHIITAKE MUSHROOM

Other names: forest mushroom, hua gu, lentinula, pasania fungus, snake butter

SUMMARY: Shiitake mushrooms have been used as a food and medicine for thousands of years in Asia. Shiitake mushrooms and lentinan, a polysaccharide isolated from the mushrooms, have possible anti-bacterial, anti-viral, cancer-fighting, and anti-hypercholesterolemic effects in *in vitro* and animal studies; human clinical data are limited. Shiitake mushrooms and lentinan stimulate T cells and macrophages. These immune-stimulating effects pose theoretical risks in MS and may decrease the effectiveness of immune-modulating and immune-suppressing medications.

References and additional reading:

Chang R. Functional properties of edible mushrooms. *Nutr Rev* 1996;1:S91–S93.

Duke JA, Bogenschutz-Godwin MJ, duCellier J, Duke P-AK. *Handbook of Medicinal Herbs.* 2nd ed. Boca Raton, FL: CRC Press, 2002:668.

Jellin JM, Gregory PJ, Batz F, et al. *Pharmacist's Letter/Prescriber's Letter Natural Medicines Comprehensive Database.* 4th ed. Stockton, CA: Therapeutic Research Faculty, 2002:1147–1148.

Peirce A. *Practical Guide to Natural Medicines*. New York: The Stonesong Press, 1999:599–600.

SIBERIAN GINSENG

Other names: ci wu jia, devil's bush, devil's shrub, eleuthera, eleuthero, *Eleutherococcus senticosus*, shigoka, thorny bearer of free berries, touch-me-not, untouchable, ussuri, ussurian thorny pepperbrush, wild pepper

SUMMARY: Siberian ginseng, which is different from American ginseng and Asian ginseng, contains eleutherosides that may have antioxidant, anti-cancer, and anti-platelet effects. Siberian ginseng is claimed to be effective for fatigue and many other conditions; clinical trials do not demonstrate definite beneficial effects for fatigue or any other condition. In fact, Siberian ginseng may cause sedation, which may worsen MS fatigue or increase the sedating effects of medications. Also, it stimulates T cells. These immune-stimulating effects pose theoretical risks in MS and may decrease the effectiveness of immune-modulating and immune-suppressing medications.

Additional information:

Dosage: 500–2000 mg P.O. daily

Contraindications and warnings: mania; schizophrenia; cardiovascular disease (palpitations, tachycardia, hypertension); rheumatic heart disease (pericardial pain); hormone-sensitive cancer (estrogenic activity); pregnancy and lactation (insufficient information)

Major interactions: sedating medications (increased sedative effect); anticoagulant and antiplatelet medications; insulin and oral hypoglycemic drugs (hypoglycemia)

Main side effects: generally well tolerated; fatigue; sciatic nerve irritation; muscle spasms; irritability; anxiety; mastalgia; hypertension; diarrhea

References and additional reading:

Bohn B, Nebe CT, Birr C. Flow-cytometric studies with *Eleutherococcus senticosus* extract as an immunomodulatory agent. *Arzneimittelforchung* 1987;37: 1193–1196.

Fetrow CW, Avila JR. *Professional's Handbook of Complementary & Alternative Medicines*. 2nd ed. Springhouse, PA: Springhouse Corp, 2001:342–345.

Fragakis AS. *The Health Professional's Guide to Popular Dietary Supplements*. 2nd ed. Chicago, IL: American Dietetic Association, 2003:211–221.

Jellin JM, Gregory PJ, Batz F, et al. *Pharmacist's Letter/Prescriber's Letter Natural Medicines Comprehensive Database*. 4th ed. Stockton, CA: Therapeutic Research Faculty, 2002:597–599.

Newall CA, Anderson LA, Phillipson JD. *Herbal Medicines: A Guide for Health-Care Professionals.* London: The Pharmaceutical Press, 1996:141–144.

SPIRULINA

Other names: AFA, BGA, blue-green algae, cyanobacteria, dihe, super seaweed, superfood, tecuitlatl

SUMMARY: Spirulina is claimed to be effective for treating MS and fatigue. The basis for this claim is not clear. There are no published clinical trials that demonstrate that spirulina is an effective therapy for MS or fatigue. Spirulina contains vitamin B12, but most MS patients have normal vitamin B12 levels, vitamin B12 has not been shown to be an effective MS therapy, and the vitamin B12 in spirulina may not be biologically active (see vitamin B12). Some spirulina products contain gamma-linolenic acid (GLA), an omega-6 polyunsaturated fatty acid (PUFA) that is also found in evening primrose oil, borage seed oil, and black currant seed oil. Clinical trials indicate that supplements of linoleic acid, another omega-6 PUFA, may mildly decrease relapse severity in MS (see Appendix I). As a source of GLA, spirulina products may not be reliable since the GLA content is variable. Activation of T cells and macrophages has been associated with spirulina; these effects may pose theoretical risks in MS and may decrease the effectiveness of immune-modulating and immune-suppressing medications. Non-contaminated spirulina products are usually well tolerated. However, some spirulina products may be contaminated with heavy metals, microbes, and microcystins. Microcystins may cause nausea, vomiting, hepatic toxicity, and death. The safety of long-term spirulina use is not known.

References and additional reading:

Bowling AC. *Alternative Medicine and Multiple Sclerosis.* New York: Demos Medical Publishing, Inc., 2001:115–116.

Bowling AC, Stewart TM. Current complementary and alternative therapies for multiple sclerosis. *Curr Treat Options Neurol* 2003;5:55–68.

Fetrow CW, Avila JR. *Professional's Handbook of Complementary & Alternative Medicines.* 2nd ed. Springhouse, PA: Springhouse Corp, 2001:735–738.

Fragakis AS. *The Health Professional's Guide to Popular Dietary Supplements.* 2nd ed. Chicago, IL: American Dietetic Association, 2003:377–382.

Hayashi O, Katoh T, Okuwaki Y. Enhancement of antibody production in mice by dietary *Spirulina platensis. J Nutr Sci Vitaminol* 1994;40:431–441.

Jellin JM, Gregory PJ, Batz F, et al. *Pharmacist's Letter/Prescriber's Letter Natural Medicines Comprehensive Database.* 4th ed. Stockton, CA: Therapeutic Research Faculty, 2002:198–199.

Qureshi MA, Ali RA. *Spirulina platensis* exposure enhances macrophage phagocytic function in cats. *Immunopharmacol Immunotoxicol* 1996;18:457–463.

STINGING NETTLE

Other names: common nettle, nettle, ortie, urtica, urticae herba et folium

SUMMARY: Stinging nettle is claimed to be an effective therapy for MS, urinary tract infections (UTIs), and many other conditions. However, there are no clinical studies of its effects on MS, and, due to its immune-stimulating effects, it poses theoretical risks in MS and may decrease the effectiveness of immune-modulating and immune-suppressing medications. In addition, stinging nettle has sedating properties that may worsen MS fatigue or increase the sedating effects of medications.

References and additional reading:

Fetrow CW, Avila JR. *Professional's Handbook of Complementary & Alternative Medicines.* 2nd ed. Springhouse, PA: Springhouse Corp, 2001:540–542.

Galelli A, Truffa-Bachi P. *Urtica dioica* agglutinin. A superantigenic lectin from stinging nettle rhizome. *J Immunol* 1993;151:1821–1831.

Jellin JM, Gregory PJ, Batz F, et al. *Pharmacist's Letter/Prescriber's Letter Natural Medicines Comprehensive Database.* 4th ed. Stockton, CA: Therapeutic Research Faculty, 2002:1188–1190.

Le Moal MA, Colle JH, Galelli A, et al. Mouse T-lymphocyte activation by *Urtica dioica* agglutinin. II. Original pattern of cell activation and cytokine production induced by UDA. *Res Immunol* 1992;143:701–709.

Peirce A. *Practical Guide to Natural Medicines.* New York: The Stonesong Press, 1999:454–457.

SUNFLOWER SEED OIL

Other names: corona solis, marigold of Peru

SUMMARY: Sunflower seed oil, like safflower seed oil, contains relatively high concentrations of linoleic acid (LA), an omega-six polyunsaturated fatty acid (PUFA). Controlled clinical trials indicate that LA supplementation may mildly decrease relapse severity and disease progression in relapsing-remitting MS (see Appendix I). Most of the LA supplementation trials have used sunflower seed oil. It has been argued that gamma-linolenic acid (GLA), another omega-6 PUFA found in evening primrose oil, borage seed oil, and black currant seed oil, may be a more physiologically useful PUFA than LA. If PUFA supplements are consumed on a regular basis, vitamin E supplements (0.6–0.9 IU of vitamin E/g PUFA) should be taken to prevent vitamin E deficiency.

Additional information:

Dosage: in studies of relapsing-remitting MS, daily doses of 17–23 g of sunflower seed oil P.O. were used

Contraindications and warnings: allergy to Asteraceae/Compositae family; pregnancy and lactation (insufficient information)

Major interactions: none known

Main side effects: usually well tolerated; the safety of long-term use of high doses is not known; since supplementation with PUFAs may produce vitamin E deficiency, supplementation with vitamin E may be necessary (0.6–0.9 IU of vitamin E/g PUFA)

References and additional reading:

Bates D, Fawcett P, Shaw D, et al. Polyunsaturated fatty acids in treatment of acute remitting multiple sclerosis. *Br Med J* 1978;2:1390–1391.

Bates D, Fawcett P, Shaw D, et al. Trial of polyunsaturated fatty acids in non-relapsing multiple sclerosis. *Br Med J* 1977;2:932–933.

Bowling AC. *Alternative Medicine and Multiple Sclerosis.* New York: Demos Medical Publishing, Inc., 2001:74–90.

Bowling AC, Stewart TM. Current complementary and alternative therapies for multiple sclerosis. *Curr Treat Options Neurol* 2003;5:55–68.

Duke JA, Bogenschutz-Godwin MJ, duCellier J, Duke P-AK. *Handbook of Medicinal Herbs.* 2nd ed. Boca Raton, FL: CRC Press, 2002:668.

Jellin JM, Gregory PJ, Batz F, et al. *Pharmacist's Letter/Prescriber's Letter Natural Medicines Comprehensive Database.* 4th ed. Stockton, CA: Therapeutic Research Faculty; 2002:1200.

Dworkin R, Bates D, Millar J, et al. Linoleic acid and multiple sclerosis: a reanalysis of three double-blind trials. *Neurol* 1984;34:1441–1445.

Millar J, Zilkha K, Langman M, et al. Double-blind trial of linoleate supplementation of the diet in multiple sclerosis. *Br Med J* 1973;1:765–768.

Paty D. Double-blind trial of linoleic acid in multiple sclerosis. *Arch Neurol* 1983;40:693–694.

THIAMINE: see "vitamin B1"

THREONINE

Other names: none

SUMMARY: Threonine is a potential amino acid precursor for glycine biosynthesis in the spinal cord. Through its conversion to glycine, threonine, which crosses the blood–brain barrier, could decrease spasticity by increasing glycinergic inhibitory signals in the motor reflex arc in the spinal cord. Two studies of MS patients found that threonine at doses of 6.0 or 7.5 g daily mildly decreased signs of spasticity by clinical examination. However, there was little or no symptomatic improvement noted by patients or physicians. There is limited safety information about supplementation with threonine; in the two short-term MS studies (two weeks and eight weeks), threonine was well tolerated.

References and additional reading:

Hauser SL, Doolittle TH, Lopez-Bresnahan M, et al. An antispasticity effect of threonine in multiple sclerosis. *Arch Neurol* 1992;49:923–926.

Lee A, Patterson V. A double-blind study of L-threonine in patients with spinal spasticity. *Acta Neurol Scand* 1993;88:334–338.

THUNDER GOD VINE

Other names: hyang-t'eng ken, lei gong teng, lei-kung t'eng, taso-ho-hua, threewingnut, *Tripterygium wilfordii*, yellow vine

SUMMARY: This Chinese herb contains several compounds with immunosuppressive effects. In EAE, disease severity is decreased by treatment with thunder god vine. One clinical trial of thunder god vine treatment in 10 MS patients in China found "significant improvement" in eight patients and mild improvement in two patients. Preliminary studies suggest beneficial effects in rheumatoid arthritis and systemic lupus erythematosus. Thunder god vine may produce serious side effects, including gastrointestinal upset, infertility, lymphocyte suppression, skin reactions, and amenorrhea. There is one case of leukopenia, renal failure, hypotension, and death that occurred three days after ingesting thunder god vine in a young man with pre-existing heart disease. Further study of this herb in MS would be worthwhile.

References and additional reading:

Bruneton J. *Toxic Plants Dangerous to Humans and Animals.* Paris: Lavoisier Publishing Inc.; 1999:229–230.

Bowling AC. *Alternative Medicine and Multiple Sclerosis*. New York: Demos Medical Publishing, Inc.; 2001:32–35.

Ho LJ, Chang DM, Chang JL, et al. Mechanism of immunosuppression of the antirheumatic herb TWHf in human T cells. *J Rheumatol* 1999;26:14–24.

Jellin JM, Gregory PJ, Batz F, et al. *Pharmacist's Letter/Prescriber's Letter Natural Medicines Comprehensive Database*. 4th ed. Stockton, CA: Therapeutic Research Faculty; 2002:1232–1233.

Yi S, Xioayan L. A review on traditional Chinese medicine in prevention and treatment of multiple sclerosis. *J Trad Chin Med* 1999;19:65–73.

Zhang L-H, Huang Y, Wang L-W, et al. Several compounds from Chinese traditional and herbal medicine as immunomodulators. *Phytother Res* 1995;9:315–322.

TRIPTERYGIUM WILFORDII: see "thunder god vine"

UVA URSI: see "bearberry"

VALERIAN

Other names: all-heal, amantilla, baldrian, garden heliotrope, herba benedicta, phu germanicum, setwall, *Valeriana officinalis*

SUMMARY: This herb may be effective for treating insomnia. Clinical trials of valerian treatment for insomnia have been of variable quality (short duration, small sample sizes, ill-defined patient groups). Further studies are needed. It may take 2–4 weeks to obtain the therapeutic effect. Valerian is also sometimes suggested as a therapy for depression, anxiety, and spasticity, but clinical trials for these conditions are limited in quality and number. Valerian is usually well tolerated. In the United States, it has received generally regarded as safe (GRAS) status. No major adverse effects have been reported in over 12,000 patients treated in trials that lasted up to 28 days. The safety of long-term use is not known. It has sedative effects that may worsen MS fatigue and may increase the sedating effects of medications.

Additional information:

Dosage: 400–900 mg of valerian extract P.O. 1/2–2 hours before bedtime; for tea, 2–3 g (1 tsp) of crude dried herb P.O. several times daily; 3–5 ml (1/2–1 tsp) of tincture P.O. several times daily

Contraindications and warnings: liver disease due to risk of liver toxicity; pregnancy and lactation (insufficient information)

Major interactions: sedating medications (excessive sedation); may inhibit cytochrome P450 3A4 and may theoretically increase levels of drugs metabolized by this enzyme (including lovastatin, ketoconazole, itraconazole, fexofenadine, triazolam, and others)

Main side effects: generally well tolerated; sedation; possibly morning drowsiness; headache; excitability; insomnia; possible benzodiazepine-like withdrawal reaction after discontinuing use of high doses or use for extended time periods—as a result, the doses should be tapered before discontinuing; possible rare hepatotoxicity; constituents of valerian, valepotriates, have produced cytotoxic effects *in vitro*, but these effects are not thought to occur *in vivo*

References and additional reading:

Bowling AC. *Alternative Medicine and Multiple Sclerosis.* New York: Demos Medical Publishing, Inc., 2001:116–117.

Fetrow CW, Avila JR. *Professional's Handbook of Complementary & Alternative Medicines.* 2nd ed. Springhouse, PA: Springhouse Corp, 2001:783–785.

Fragakis AS. *The Health Professional's Guide to Popular Dietary Supplements.* 2nd ed. Chicago, IL: American Dietetic Association, 2003:382–387.

Jellin JM, Gregory PJ, Batz F, et al. *Pharmacist's Letter/Prescriber's Letter Natural Medicines Comprehensive Database.* 4th ed. Stockton, CA: Therapeutic Research Faculty, 2002:1262–1264.

Mischoulon D, Rosenbaum JF. *Natural Medications for Psychiatric Disorders: Considering the Alternatives.* Philadelphia, PA: Lippincott Williams & Wilkins, 2002:132–146.

Russo E. *Handbook of Psychotropic Herbs: A Scientific Analysis of Herbal Remedies for Psychiatric Conditions.* New York: The Haworth Herbal Press, 2001:95–106.

Schulz V, Hänsel R, Tyler VE. *Rational Phytotherapy: A Physicians' Guide to Herbal Medicine.* 3rd ed. Berlin: Springer-Verlag, 1998:73–81.

VITAMIN A/BETA-CAROTENE

Other names: 3–dehydroretinol, antixerophthalmic vitamin, beta-carotene, dehydroretinol, retinal, retinoids, vitamin A1, vitamin A2

SUMMARY: Vitamin A, a fat-soluble vitamin, is actually a family of structurally related molecules known as retinoids. Carotenoids, including beta-carotene, are vitamin A precursors that are found in fruits and vegetables. Beta-carotene and vitamin A have many biological actions, including antioxidant and immunologic effects. Several studies have evaluated whether supplementation with beta-carotene in humans has immune-modulating or immune-stimulating effects; variable findings have been reported and some studies have not found any effect on T cell function. Retinoids decrease disease severity in experimental allergic encephalomyelitis (EAE). One retinoid, all-*trans* retinoic acid, decreases lymphocyte proliferation and increases the ability of interferon beta-1b to augment T suppressor cell function. Further studies are needed to determine the effect of beta-carotene and vitamin A on MS and the activity of immune-suppressing and immune-modulating drugs.

Additional information:

Dosage: for adults, the RDAs for vitamin A are 2300 IU (700 mcg) for women and 3000 IU (900 mcg) for men; the Tolerable Upper Intake Level (UL) for vitamin A is 10,000 IU daily for men and women; there is no established UL for carotenoids

Contraindications and warnings: angioplasty (decreased vascular remodeling); male smokers (increased risk of lung cancer, myocardial infarction, and intracerebral hemorrhage with beta-carotene supplements); asbestos workers (increased risk of lung cancer with beta-carotene supplements); liver disease (increased risk of hypervitaminosis A and hepatotoxicity); osteoporosis and osteopenia (high doses may increase the risk of osteoporosis)

Major interactions: minocycline and vitamin A (pseudotumor cerebri); HMG-CoA reductase inhibitors and oral contraceptives (increased blood levels of vitamin A)

Main side effects: generally well tolerated in reasonable doses; high doses (>10,000 IU daily) may produce multiple toxic effects, especially in pregnant women (birth defects); toxic effects include osteoporosis, fatigue, abdominal pain, nausea, vomiting, joint pain, muscle pain, increased intracranial pressure, pseudotumor cerebri, dizziness, visual changes, dry skin and lips, brittle nails, cirrhosis, jaundice, ascites, and increased liver function tests

References and additional reading:

Bowling AC. *Alternative Medicine and Multiple Sclerosis*. New York: Demos Medical Publishing, Inc., 2001:187–189.

Fragakis AS. *The Health Professional's Guide to Popular Dietary Supplements*. 2nd ed. Chicago, IL: American Dietetic Association, 2003:392–405.

Grimble RF. Effect of antioxidative vitamins on immune function with clinical applications. *Int J Vit Res* 1997;67:312–320.

Harbige LS. Nutrition and immunity with emphasis on infection and autoimmune disease. *Nutr Health* 1996;10:285–312.

Jellin JM, Gregory PJ, Batz F, et al. *Pharmacist's Letter/Prescriber's Letter Natural Medicines Comprehensive Database*. 4th ed. Stockton, CA: Therapeutic Research Faculty, 2002:131–134.

Lovett-Racke AE, Racke MK. Retinoic acid promotes the development of Th2–like human myelin basic protein-reactive T cells. *Cell Immunol* 2002;215:54–60.

Massacesi L, Abbamoudi AL, Biorgi C, et al. Suppression of experimental allergic encephalomyelitis by retinoic acid. *J Neurol Sci* 1987;80:55–64.

Qu ZX, Pliskin N, Jensen MW, et al. Etritinate augments interferon beta-1b effects on suppressor cells in multiple sclerosis. *Arch Neurol* 2001;58:87–90.

VITAMIN B1/THIAMINE

Other names: antiberiberi factor, antineuritic factor, anurine, B complex vitamin, thiamine

SUMMARY: Thiamine has no clear relevance to MS. It is sometimes claimed to be effective for treating fatigue in the general population. However, it has not been shown to be an effective treatment for fatigue. For adults, the RDA is 1.1 mg for women and 1.2 mg for men. There is not an established Tolerable Upper Intake Level (UL) for thiamine.

References and additional reading:

Fragakis AS. *The Health Professional's Guide to Popular Dietary Supplements*. 2nd ed. Chicago, IL: American Dietetic Association, 2003:405–409.

Jellin JM, Gregory PJ, Batz F, et al. *Pharmacist's Letter/Prescriber's Letter Natural Medicines Comprehensive Database*. 4th ed. Stockton, CA: Therapeutic Research Faculty, 2002:1230–1232.

VITAMIN B2/RIBOFLAVIN

Other names: B complex vitamin, flavin, lactoflavin, riboflavin, vitamin G

SUMMARY: Riboflavin, which may be effective for migraine prevention, has no apparent applications to MS. For adults, the RDA is 1.3 mg for men and 1.1 mg for women. A Tolerable Upper Intake Level (UL) has not been determined.

References and additional reading:

Fragakis AS. *The Health Professional's Guide to Popular Dietary Supplements*. 2nd ed. Chicago, IL: American Dietetic Association, 2003:410–412.

Jellin JM, Gregory PJ, Batz F, et al. *Pharmacist's Letter/Prescriber's Letter Natural Medicines Comprehensive Database*. 4th ed. Stockton, CA: Therapeutic Research Faculty, 2002:1081–1083.

VITAMIN B3/NIACIN

Other names: 3–pyridine carboxamine, anti-blacktongue factor, antipellagra factor, B complex vitamin, niacin, niacinamide, nicotinic acid, pellagra preventing factor, vitamin PP

SUMMARY: Niacin has no apparent relevance to MS. Niacin includes nicotinic acid (nicotinate) and nicotinamide (niacinamide). The RDAs for niacin are 16 mg for adult men and 14 mg for adult women. Niacin may produce nausea, flushing, hepatotoxicity, and hyperglycemia, especially in doses that exceed the Tolerable Upper Intake Level (UL) of 35 mg.

References and additional reading:

Bowling AC. *Alternative Medicine and Multiple Sclerosis.* New York: Demos Medical Publishing, Inc., 2001:194.

Fragakis AS. *The Health Professional's Guide to Popular Dietary Supplements.* 2nd ed. Chicago, IL: American Dietetic Association, 2003:412–418.

Jellin JM, Gregory PJ, Batz F, et al. *Pharmacist's Letter/Prescriber's Letter Natural Medicines Comprehensive Database.* 4th ed. Stockton, CA: Therapeutic Research Faculty, 2002:919–923.

VITAMIN B6/PYRIDOXINE

Other names: adermine hydrochloride, B complex vitamin, pyridoxal, pyridoxamine, pyridoxine

SUMMARY: There is no clear relevance of pyridoxine to MS. The RDA is 1.3 mg for men and women who are 19–50 years old, 1.5 mg for women older than 50 years, and 1.7 mg for men older than 50 years. Pyridoxine deficiency and excess (>50 mg daily) may cause polyneuropathy. Pyridoxine has immune-stimulating effects. Due to these effects, the use of pyridoxine supplements, especially in high doses or for prolonged periods of time, poses theoretical risks in MS and could decrease the effectiveness of immune-modulating and immune-suppressing medications.

References and additional reading:

Fragakis AS. *The Health Professional's Guide to Popular Dietary Supplements.* 2nd ed. Chicago, IL: American Dietetic Association, 2003:418–426.

Grimble RF. Effect of antioxidative vitamins on immune function with clinical applications. *Int J Vit Res* 1997;67:312–320.

Jellin JM, Gregory PJ, Batz F, et al. *Pharmacist's Letter/Prescriber's Letter Natural Medicines Comprehensive Database.* 4th ed. Stockton, CA: Therapeutic Research Faculty, 2002:1051–1055.

VITAMIN B12

Other names: B-12, B complex vitamin, cobamin, cobalamin, cyanocobalamin, methylcobalamin

SUMMARY: Vitamin B12 supplements are sometimes claimed to be effective for treating MS. However, there are no studies to support the widespread use of vitamin B12 supplements in MS patients. A small fraction of MS patients may have vitamin B12 deficiency. Supplementation is recommended in these patients. For MS patients who do not have vitamin B12 deficiency, there is no evidence that vitamin B12 supplementation is beneficial. One small six-month study of high-dose vitamin B12 supplementation (60 mg P.O. daily for six months) in six progressive MS patients found that the level of disability was stable or worsened. "Improvement" in evoked potentials was noted in some treated patients; the significance of this finding is not clear.

Additional information:

Dosage: for vitamin B12 deficiency, 1 mg I.M. daily for one week, 1 mg I.M. weekly for one month, then 1 mg I.M. monthly for life; for vitamin B12 deficiency, oral vitamin B12 supplements (100–1,000 mcg P.O. daily) may also be effective; for use as a dietary supplement, 1–25 mcg P.O. daily; the RDA for adults is 2.4 mcg; adverse effects have not been reported with the use of high doses; there is no established Tolerable Upper Intake Level (UL)

Contraindications and warnings: Leber's hereditary optic neuropathy

Major interactions: folic acid supplements may mask the hematologic abnormalities associated with vitamin B12 deficiency

Main side effects: usually well tolerated; diarrhea; rashes; urticaria

References and additional reading:

Bowling AC. *Alternative Medicine and Multiple Sclerosis.* New York: Demos Medical Publishing, Inc., 2001:193–194.

Bowling AC, Ibrahim R, Stewart TM. Alternative medicine and multiple sclerosis: an objective review from an American perspective. *Int J MS Care* 2000;2:14–21.

Bowling AC, Stewart TM. Current complementary and alternative therapies for multiple sclerosis. *Curr Treat Options Neurol* 2003;5:55–68.

Fragakis AS. *The Health Professional's Guide to Popular Dietary Supplements.* 2nd ed. Chicago, IL: American Dietetic Association, 2003:426–433.

Jellin JM, Gregory PJ, Batz F, et al. *Pharmacist's Letter/Prescriber's Letter Natural Medicines Comprehensive Database.* 4th ed. Stockton, CA: Therapeutic Research Faculty, 2002:1277–1280.

Reynolds E, Bottiglieri T, Laundy M, et al. Vitamin B12 metabolism in multiple sclerosis. *Arch Neurol* 1992;49:649–652.

Goodkin D, Jacobsen D, Galvez N, et al. Serum cobalamin deficiency is uncommon in multiple sclerosis. *Arch Neurol* 1994;51:1110–1114.

Kira J, Tobimatus S, Goto I. Vitamin B12 metabolism and massive-dose methyl vitamin B12 therapy in Japanese patients with multiple sclerosis. *Int Med* 1994;33:82–86.

Rowland L. *Merritt's Neurology-10th ed.* Philadelphia, PA: Lippincott Williams & Wilkins 2000, 898.

VITAMIN C

Other names: antiscorbutic vitamin, ascorbic acid

SUMMARY: For several reasons, vitamin C is sometimes recommended as a therapy for MS. First, MS patients may be prone to urinary tract infections (UTIs) and there is suggestive evidence that vitamin C may prevent UTIs. However, for UTI prevention with dietary supplements, there is better evidence for cranberry than for vitamin C. Another effect of vitamin C that is of potential relevance to MS is that it may mildly decrease the duration of the common cold. It is known that viral infections, such as the common cold, may precipitate MS exacerbations. Thus, a therapy that decreases the duration of the common cold could secondarily decrease the risk of an exacerbation. However, the effects of vitamin C on the common cold are equivocal, and, as noted below, vitamin C carries some theoretical risks in MS. Finally, vitamin C is also sometimes recommended for MS treatment because of its antioxidant effects. Indeed, there is suggestive evidence that free radical-induced oxidative injury is elevated in patients with MS and that oxidative damage is involved in myelin and axonal damage. However, many antioxidant compounds, including vitamin C, stimulate T cells and macrophages. Thus, vitamin C poses theoretical risks in MS and could antagonize the effects of immune-modulating and immune-suppressing medications. In a five-week study of 18 MS patients, supplementation with selenium, vitamin C, and vitamin E did not produce any significant adverse effects. Further studies are needed to determine the safety and efficacy, if any, of vitamin C and other antioxidants in MS. Until more information is available, it may be most reasonable for MS patients to obtain antioxidant compounds through dietary sources such as fruits (two to four servings daily) and vegetables (three to five servings daily). If vitamin C supplements are taken in MS, it may be best to use modest doses (90–120 mg daily).

Additional information:

Dosage: the RDAs for vitamin C are 75 mg for women (except during pregnancy and lactation) and 90 mg for men; for smokers, the RDA is 35 mg or greater; for treating the common cold, doses of 1–3 g P.O. daily have been used; doses that exceed the Tolerable Upper Intake Level (UL) of 2000 mg daily should be avoided

Contraindications and warnings: angioplasty (decreased vascular remodeling); history of kidney stones (increased risk of oxalate stone formation, especially with doses greater than 1000 mg daily)

Major interactions: anticoagulant medications (decreased effectiveness)

Main side effects: usually well tolerated in reasonable doses; increased risk of side effects with higher doses; possible side effects include nausea, abdominal cramping, diarrhea, fatigue, headache, insomnia, hyperoxaluria, kidney stones (in patients with a history of kidney stones)

References and additional reading:

Bowling A, Beal M. Bioenergetic and oxidative stress in neurodegenerative diseases. *Life Sci* 1995;56:1151–1171.

Bowling AC, Ibrahim R, Stewart TM. Alternative medicine and multiple sclerosis: an objective review from an American perspective. *Int J MS Care* 2000;2:14–21.

Bowling AC, Stewart TM. Current complementary and alternative therapies for multiple sclerosis. *Curr Treat Options Neurol* 2003;5:55–68.

Castello T, Girona L, Gomez MR, et al. The possible value of ascorbic acid as a prophylactic agent for urinary tract infection. *Spinal Cord* 1996;34:592–593.

Fragakis AS. *The Health Professional's Guide to Popular Dietary Supplements.* 2nd ed. Chicago, IL: American Dietetic Association, 2003:433–445.

Greco A, Minghetti L, Sette G, et al. Cerebrospinal fluid isoprostane shows oxidative stress in patients with multiple sclerosis. *Neurol* 1999;53:1876–1879.

Grimble R. Effect of antioxidative vitamins on immune function with clinical applications. *Int J Vitam Nutr Res* 1997;67:312–320.

Hooper D, Bagasra O, Marini J, et al. Prevention of experimental allergic encephalomyelitis by targeting nitric oxide and peroxynitrite: implications for the treatment of multiple sclerosis. *Proc Natl Acad Sci USA* 1997;94:2528–2533.

Jellin JM, Gregory PJ, Batz F, et al. *Pharmacist's Letter/Prescriber's Letter Natural Medicines Comprehensive Database.* 4th ed. Stockton, CA: Therapeutic Research Faculty, 2002:1280–1286.

Mai J, Sorenson P, Hansen J. High dose antioxidant supplementation to MS patients: effects on glutathione peroxidase, clinical safety, and absorption of selenium. *Biol Trace Elem Res* 1990;24:109–117.

Trapp B, Ransohoff R, Fisher E, et al. Neurodegeneration in multiple sclerosis: relationship to neurological disability. *Neuroscientist* 1999;5:1–7.

VITAMIN D

Other names: alfacalcidol, calcifediol, calcipotriene, calcitriol, cholecalciferol, ergocalciferol, paricalcitol

SUMMARY: Vitamin D is considered a hormone and a vitamin. It acts primarily to maintain calcium homeostasis. There are two ways in which vitamin D is relevant to MS. First, MS patients may be especially prone to osteopenia and osteoporosis. These conditions are probably underdiagnosed and undertreated in MS patients. Vitamin D, calcium, and other therapies are important in preventing and treating decreased bone density. Another MS-relevant aspect of vitamin D is that it is mildly immunosuppressive. Vitamin D decreases the production of proinflammatory cytokines and inhibits lymphocyte proliferation. In EAE, disease severity is decreased by vitamin D supplementation and increased by vitamin D deficiency. There are limited clinical trial studies of vitamin D treatment in MS patients. In one older uncontrolled study, attack rate was decreased in 10 MS patients who were treated with supplements of magnesium, calcium, and cod-liver oil, which contains vitamin D, vitamin A, and omega-3 fatty acids. The preliminary report of a more recent small, short-term study indicates that treatment of 11 MS patients with 19–nor, a vitamin D analog, did not significantly affect disease activity on the basis of attack rate or MRI measures. Further studies of the effects of vitamin D on MS are underway.

Additional information:

Dosage: the Adequate Intake (AI) for vitamin D is 200 IU for adults less than 50 years, 400 IU for adults 51–70 years, and 600 IU for adults greater than 70 years; doses greater than the Tolerable Upper Intake Level (UL) of 2000 IU should be avoided; taking vitamin D supplements along with a high intake of vitamin D-rich foods, such as fish and fortified milk, increases the risk of vitamin D toxicity

Contraindications and warnings: hypercalcemia; sarcoidosis; hypoparathyroidism; renal disease

Major interactions: cardiac glycosides (hypercalcemia-induced arrhythmias)

Main side effects: generally well tolerated in reasonable doses; high doses of vitamin D may cause hypercalcemia, nausea, vomiting, abdominal cramps, fatigue, muscle and bone pain, renal insufficiency, and hypertension

References and additional reading:

Bowling AC, Ibrahim R, Stewart TM. Alternative medicine and multiple sclerosis: an objective review from an American perspective. *Int J MS Care* 2000;2:14–21.

Bowling AC, Stewart TM. Current complementary and alternative therapies for multiple sclerosis. *Curr Treat Options Neurol* 2003;5:55–68.

Cantorna M, Hayes C, DeLuca H. 1,25–dihydroxyvitamin D3 reversibly blocks the progression of relapsing encephalomyelitis, a model of multiple sclerosis. *Proc Natl Acad Sci USA* 1996;93:7861–7864.

Cantorna M, Humpal-Winter J, DeLuca H. In vivo upregulation of interleukin-4 is one mechanism underlying the immunoregulatory effects of 1,25–dihydrox-yvitamin D3. *Arch Biochem Biophys* 2000;377:135–138.

Fleming J, Hummel A, Beinlich B, et al. Vitamin D treatment of relapsing-remitting multiple sclerosis (RRMS): a MRI-based pilot study. *Neurol* 2000;54:A338.

Fragakis AS. *The Health Professional's Guide to Popular Dietary Supplements*. 2nd ed. Chicago, IL: American Dietetic Association, 2003:445–451.

Herndon R, Mohandas N: Osteoporosis in multiple sclerosis: a frequent, serious, and under-recognized problem. *Int J MS Care* 2000;2(2):5.

Jellin JM, Gregory PJ, Batz F, et al. *Pharmacist's Letter/Prescriber's Letter Natural Medicines Comprehensive Database*. 4th ed. Stockton, CA: Therapeutic Research Faculty, 2002:1296–1290.

Smeltzer S, Zimmerman V, Capriotti T, et al. Osteoporosis risk factors and bone mineral density in women with MS. *Int J MS Care* 2000;4:17–23,29.

Van Etten E, Brainistreanu D, Verstuyf A, et al. Analogs of I,25–dihydroxyvitamin D3 as dose-reducing agents for classical immunosuppressants. *Transplantation* 2000;69:1932–1942.

VITAMIN E

Other names: alpha-tocopherol, tocopherol

SUMMARY: Vitamin E is a fat-soluble antioxidant vitamin that exists in multiple forms. Alpha-tocopherol is the most abundant and most active form of vitamin E. Vitamin E has relevance to MS in two main areas. First, vitamin E is sometimes suggested as an MS treatment because of its antioxidant properties. There is some evidence that free radical-induced oxidative injury is elevated in patients with MS and that oxidative injury is involved in myelin and axonal damage. However, many antioxidant compounds, including vitamin E, activate macrophages and T cells. Consequently, vitamin E poses theoretical risks in MS and could antagonize the effects of immune-modulating and immune-suppressing medications. A five-week study of 18 MS patients found that supplementation with vitamin E, vitamin C, and selenium did not produce significant adverse effects. Further studies are needed to evaluate the safety and efficacy of vitamin E and other antioxidants in MS. Until more information is available, it may be most reasonable for MS patients to obtain antioxidant compounds through dietary sources such as fruits (two to four servings daily) and vegetables (three to five servings daily). If MS patients do take vitamin E supplements, it may be best to use modest doses (100–400 IU daily). The other MS-relevant aspect of vitamin E is for patients who consume diets or supplements high in polyunsaturated fatty acids (PUFAs) for possible disease-modifying effects. In this situation, vitamin E supplementation (0.6–0.9 IU of vitamin E/g PUFA) is needed to prevent vitamin E deficiency (see sunflower seed oil).

Additional information:

Dosage: the RDA for adults for vitamin E is 15 mg from food (alpha-tocopherol), which is equivalent to 22 IU of natural vitamin E or 33 IU of synthetic vitamin E; as noted above, if vitamin E supplements are taken by MS patients due to a high PUFA diet or for other reasons, it may be best to use modest doses (100–400 IU daily); avoid daily doses greater than the Tolerable Upper Intake Level (UL) of 1000 mg (equivalent to 1100 IU of synthetic vitamin E or 1500 IU of natural vitamin E); for conversions with lower, nontoxic doses, 1 mg of alpha-tocopherol = 1.5 IU of natural vitamin E = 2.2 IU of synthetic vitamin E

Contraindications and warnings: angioplasty (decreased vascular remodeling); retinitis pigmentosa (accelerated visual decline with synthetic vitamin E supplements); vitamin K deficiency (worsened coagulation defects)

Major interactions: anticoagulant and antiplatelet medications (increased bleeding risk)

Main side effects: usually well tolerated in reasonable doses; increased risk of bleeding, especially with doses in excess of the UL; rarely nausea, diarrhea, fatigue, stomach cramps, blurred vision, and headache

References and additional reading:

Bowling AC. *Alternative Medicine and Multiple Sclerosis.* New York: Demos Medical Publishing, Inc., 2001:187–190.

Bowling AC, Stewart TM. Current complementary and alternative therapies for multiple sclerosis. *Curr Treat Options Neurol* 2003;5:55–68.

Fragakis AS. *The Health Professional's Guide to Popular Dietary Supplements.* 2nd ed. Chicago, IL: American Dietetic Association, 2003:451–467.

Harris P, Embree N. Quantitative consideration of the effect of polyunsaturated fatty acid content of the diet upon the requirements for vitamin E. *Am J Clin Nutr* 1963;13:385–392.

Jellin JM, Gregory PJ, Batz F, et al. *Pharmacist's Letter/Prescriber's Letter Natural Medicines Comprehensive Database.* 4th ed. Stockton, CA: Therapeutic Research Faculty, 2002:1290–1298.

VITAMIN K

Other names: menadione (vitamin K3); phytonadione (vitamin K1)

SUMMARY: Vitamin K, derived from the German term *Koagulations-vitamin*, refers to a group of related compounds that play an important role in coagulation. In the United States, vitamin K1 is the only form of vitamin K available. There is no known relevance of vitamin K to MS. Vitamin K may decrease the effectiveness of warfarin (Coumadin®). The RDAs for vitamin K are 90 mcg for women and 120 mcg for men.

References and additional reading:

Jellin JM, Gregory PJ, Batz F, et al. *Pharmacist's Letter/Prescriber's Letter Natural Medicines Comprehensive Database.* 4th ed. Stockton, CA: Therapeutic Research Faculty, 2002:1298–1301.

WILD CARROT

Other names: beesnest plant, bird's nest root, devil's plague, mother's dye, Queen Anne's lace

SUMMARY: Wild carrot has sedating properties that may worsen MS fatigue or increase the sedating effects of medications.

References and additional reading:

Fetrow CW, Avila JR. *Professional's Handbook of Complementary & Alternative Medicines.* 2nd ed. Springhouse, PA: Springhouse Corp, 2001:643–645.

Jellin JM, Gregory PJ, Batz F, et al. *Pharmacist's Letter/Prescriber's Letter Natural Medicines Comprehensive Database.* 4th ed. Stockton, CA: Therapeutic Research Faculty, 2002:1328–1329.

WILD LETTUCE

Other names: acrid lettuce, bitter lettuce, green endive, lettuce opium, poison lettuce

SUMMARY: Wild lettuce has sedating effects that may worsen MS fatigue or increase the sedating actions of medications. Also, this herb may increase the risk of bleeding when used concomitantly with antiplatelet or anticoagulant medications.

References and additional reading:

Fetrow CW, Avila JR. *Professional's Handbook of Complementary & Alternative Medicines.* 2nd ed. Springhouse, PA: Springhouse Corp, 2001:804–806.

Jellin JM, Gregory PJ, Batz F, et al. *Pharmacist's Letter/Prescriber's Letter Natural Medicines Comprehensive Database.* 4th ed. Stockton, CA: Therapeutic Research Faculty, 2002:1332–1334.

WILLOW

Other names: basket willow, bay willow, black willow, crack willow, purple osier willow, violet willow, white willow

SUMMARY: This herb, which is used primarily for viral syndromes, myalgias, and other inflammatory conditions, contains salicylates that may increase the toxicity of methotrexate and may increase the risk of bleeding when taken concomitantly with antiplatelet or anticoagulant medications.

References and additional reading:

Fetrow CW, Avila JR. *Professional's Handbook of Complementary & Alternative Medicines.* 2nd ed. Springhouse, PA: Springhouse Corp, 2001:808–811.

Jellin JM, Gregory PJ, Batz F, et al. *Pharmacist's Letter/Prescriber's Letter Natural Medicines Comprehensive Database.* 4th ed. Stockton, CA: Therapeutic Research Faculty, 2002:1339–1340.

WINTERGREEN OIL

Other names: boxberry, Canada tea, checkerberry, deerberry, ground berry, hilberry, partridge berry, spiceberry, teaberry, wax cluster

SUMMARY: This herb, which should not be taken orally, contains salicylates that may increase the toxicity of methotrexate and may increase the risk of bleeding when taken concomitantly with antiplatelet or anticoagulant medications.

References and additional reading:

Fetrow CW, Avila JR. *Professional's Handbook of Complementary & Alternative Medicines.* 2nd ed. Springhouse, PA: Springhouse Corp, 2001:811–813.

Jellin JM, Gregory PJ, Batz F, et al. *Pharmacist's Letter/Prescriber's Letter Natural Medicines Comprehensive Database.* 4th ed. Stockton, CA: Therapeutic Research Faculty, 2002:1348–1349.

WOODY NIGHT SHADE

Other names: bittersweet nightshade, bittersweet, blue nightshade, deadly nightshade, fellen, fever, twig, mortal, scarlet berry, snake berry, violet bloom, woody

SUMMARY: For unclear reasons, *The Complete German Commission E Monographs*, a comprehensive German herbal medicine text, states that MS patients should not use woody nightshade, an uncommon herb.

References and additional reading:

Blumenthal M (ed.). *The Complete German Commission E Monographs: Therapeutic Guide to Herbal Medicines*. Austin: American Botanical Council, 1998:441.

Jellin JM, Gregory PJ, Batz F, et al. *Pharmacist's Letter/Prescriber's Letter Natural Medicines Comprehensive Database*. 4th ed. Stockton, CA: Therapeutic Research Faculty, 2002:158–159.

YERBA MANSA

Other names: lizard's tail, swamp root

SUMMARY: This herb has sedating properties that may worsen MS fatigue or increase the sedating effects of medications. Also, it may act as a urinary irritant.

References and additional reading:

Jellin JM, Gregory PJ, Batz F, et al. *Pharmacist's Letter/Prescriber's Letter Natural Medicines Comprehensive Database*. 4th ed. Stockton, CA: Therapeutic Research Faculty, 2002:1336–1367.

YOHIMBE

Other names: aphrodien, corynine, johimbi, yohimbehe, yohimbine

SUMMARY: Yohimbe refers to the bark from the yohimbe tree, an evergreen that is native to Zaire, Cameroon, and Gabon. Yohimbe contains yohimbine, an alkaloid, which is available by prescription. Yohimbe and yohimbine are possibly effective for treating erectile dysfunction and SSRI-induced sexual dysfunction. However, unmonitored, nonprescription use of yohimbe is not recommended due to possible serious side effects, including severe hypotension, cardiac conduction disorders, cardiac failure, and death. Other side effects include tremor, insomnia, anxiety, mania, hypertension, tachycardia, headache, nausea, and vomiting.

References and additional reading:

Fetrow CW, Avila JR. *Professional's Handbook of Complementary & Alternative Medicines*. 2nd ed. Springhouse, PA: Springhouse Corp, 2001:829–831.

Fragakis AS. *The Health Professional's Guide to Popular Dietary Supplements.* 2nd ed. Chicago, IL: American Dietetic Association, 2003:474–478.

Jellin JM, Gregory PJ, Batz F, et al. *Pharmacist's Letter/Prescriber's Letter Natural Medicines Comprehensive Database.* 4th ed. Stockton, CA: Therapeutic Research Faculty, 2002:1374–1376.

YOHIMBINE: see "yohimbe"

ZINC

Other names: zinc acetate, acexamate, zinc gluconate, zinc picolinate, zinc sulfate

SUMMARY: Zinc is a trace mineral that plays a role in many different biological processes, including immune function, carbohydrate metabolism, and protein and nucleic acid synthesis. In the 1880s, Charcot's colleagues actually used zinc phosphate as a treatment for MS. Currently, there are several MS-relevant aspects of zinc use. First, zinc is sometimes recommended for MS because it has effects on immune function. However, zinc has multiple immune system effects, including stimulation of pro-inflammatory cytokine release and T-cell proliferation. These effects carry theoretical risks in MS and could antagonize the effects of immune-modulating and immune-suppressing medications. Indeed, there are studies that raise concerns about zinc use in MS. In experimental allergic encephalomyelitis (EAE), zinc supplements may increase disease severity. In addition, a relatively high prevalence of MS was reported in workers in a zinc-related industry in New York. Finally, there is a case report of white matter lesions developing in an individual with high zinc levels (and low copper levels). Another MS-relevant aspect of zinc is in the treatment of the common cold. Zinc gluconate lozenges decrease the duration of the common cold in some, but not all, studies. Since the common cold and other viral infections may trigger MS exacerbations, decreasing the duration of these infections could be beneficial for MS patients. However, as noted, zinc carries theoretical risks in MS, and its effects on the common cold are equivocal. Zinc is also of potential relevance to MS because of its role in polyunsaturated fatty acid (PUFA) metabolism. As an MS therapy, zinc supplements are sometimes recommended in conjunction with a high PUFA diet (see sunflower seed oil) since zinc is involved in the metabolism of PUFAs. While a high PUFA diet may be beneficial, it is not clear that supplemental zinc provides any additional benefit and it actually carries theoretical risks due to immune stimulation. In conclusion, although zinc is sometimes recommended for MS, there are no strong reasons to support its use and there are theoretical risks associated with its use in MS. If MS patients use zinc, it may be best to use modest doses (10–15 mg or less daily). If high doses are taken, then copper supplements may be necessary to avoid copper deficiency.

Additional information:

Dosage: the RDA for zinc is 11 mg for men and 8 mg for women (11–12 mg during pregnancy and 12–13 mg during lactation); avoid doses above the Tolerable Upper Intake Level (UL) of 40 mg daily; to avoid copper deficiency with high zinc intake, copper supplements should be taken; cupric sulfate at doses up to 0.1 mg/kg daily have been used for treating copper deficiency (for copper, the adult RDA is 900 mcg daily and the adult Tolerable Upper Intake Level [UL] is 10 mg daily)

Contraindications and warnings: HIV infection (decreased survival); hemochromatosis

Major interactions: potassium-sparing and thiazide diuretics (increased zinc levels); tetracyclines and fluoroquinolones (decreased drug levels)

Main side effects: generally well tolerated in reasonable doses; chronic use of high doses (100–300 mg daily, but also may occur with 15–100 mg daily) may impair immune function, produce copper deficiency, and adversely affect cholesterol levels; milder side effects include unpleasant taste, mouth irritation, and nausea

References and additional reading:

Bowling AC. *Alternative Medicine and Multiple Sclerosis*. New York: Demos Medical Publishing, Inc., 2001:196–197.

Fragakis AS. *The Health Professional's Guide to Popular Dietary Supplements*. 2nd ed. Chicago, IL: American Dietetic Association, 2003:478–487.

Jellin JM, Gregory PJ, Batz F, et al. *Pharmacist's Letter/Prescriber's Letter Natural Medicines Comprehensive Database*. 4th ed. Stockton, CA: Therapeutic Research Faculty, 2002:1378–1384.

Prodan CI, Holland NR. CNS demyelination from zinc toxicity? *Neurol* 2000;54:1705.

Schiffer RB, Herndon RM, Eskin T. Effects of altered dietary trace metals upon experimental allergic encephalomyelitis. *Neuro Toxicol* 1990;11:443–450.

Stein EC, Schiffer RB, Hall WJ, et al. Multiple sclerosis and the workplace: report of an industry-based cluster. *Neurol* 1987;37:1672–1677.

Appendix I
Fatty Acids and MS

The single most well studied nonpharmaceutical intervention in MS is supplementation with polyunsaturated fatty acids (PUFAs), which include omega-3 and omega-6 fatty acids. Examples of omega-3 fatty acids include alpha linoleic acid (ALA), eicosapentaenoic acid (EPA), and docasahexanoic acid (DHA). Examples of omega-6 fatty acids include linoleic acid (LA) and gamma-linolenic acid (GLA).

There is a wide range of evidence that PUFAs may have therapeutic effects in MS. This evidence includes data from epidemiologic, immunologic, and animal model studies. Epidemiologic evidence has shown a positive association between the amount of saturated fat consumed and mortality rates from MS, and an inverse association between the ratio of polyunsaturated fats to saturated fats consumed and mortality rates from MS.[1] Many studies of PUFAs, especially omega-3 PUFAs, have demonstrated immunomodulatory effects, including decreased lymphocyte proliferation and reduced production of pro-inflammatory cytokines by lymphocytes.[2,3] PUFAs have also been studied in experimental allergic encephalomyelitis (EAE). Omega-6 fatty acids have been shown to suppress EAE.[4] There is limited and conflicting evidence regarding omega-3 fatty acids in EAE.[4]

At least six uncontrolled studies of PUFAs in MS have been reported.[5–10] In none of these was any worsening of MS observed. In most, clinical improvement was reported.

Five randomized, controlled clinical trials of PUFAs among people with relapsing-remitting MS have been reported.[11–15] Three of these involved LA and two involved a combination of EPA and DHA. In none of the three prospective LA studies was an effect on disability progression or exacerbation frequency observed.[12–14] However, all three LA studies were underpowered to detect even modest effects and, thus, the possibility that a treatment effect was missed (a Type II error) remains.[16]

In two of the three LA studies, a statistically significant reduction in exacerbation severity and duration was reported.[13,14] Interpreting these results is difficult because of the quirky scoring system used for measuring exacerbation severity and because of poor reporting. In addition, an effect on exacerbation severity is difficult to reconcile with a failure to detect an effect on exacerbation frequency.

The three prospective LA studies were later pooled and reanalyzed on the basis of post-hoc hypotheses.[17] On the basis of the post-hoc reanalysis, "patients with little or no disability at the start of the trial (Disability Status Scale [DSS] 2 or less) had a significantly smaller increase in disability than did those in the control group ($p=0.05$.)" Mean increase in disability for the LA group was 0.12, and for the control group, it was 0.81. However, the reanalysis omitted some contrary data from one of the three prospective trials, and the reported results may have statistical flaws. Given these criticisms, it may be best to view the post-hoc reanalysis as having generated an interesting, but untested, hypothesis.

One of the EPA and DHA studies was a large (312 patients) randomized, double-blind, controlled clinical trial.[11] Although no statistically significant difference was observed, there was a trend favoring the treatment group showing fewer people progressing one point on the DSS (<0.07). Sustained disability was not measured and an intent-to-treat analysis was not used. Other nonstatistically significant trends favoring the treatment group were observed. Specifically, the treatment group had fewer and shorter exacerbations than the control group.

Another small (29 patients) randomized study investigated EPA and DHA as a treatment among users of FDA-approved MS therapies. This study has been reported preliminarily.[15] Patients who had been using FDA-approved therapies for at least two months were assigned to receive either six fish oil capsules along with instructions to maintain a very low-fat diet ($<15\%$ calories from fat), or six olive oil capsules along with instructions to maintain a low-fat diet ($<30\%$ calories from fat). Those taking the fish oil capsules, but not those taking the olive oil capsules, experienced a decrease in relapse rate. Average Expanded Disability Status Scale (EDSS) scores worsened in the group taking olive oil, but not in those taking fish oil ($p=0.043$).

In none of the five prospective studies described above was safety or tolerability carefully reported. But, some sources state that LA, EPA, and DHA in reasonable doses are generally thought to be safe.[18] They are also inexpensive. Under these circumstances, a type II error may be worse than a type I error (failing to detect a true treatment effect). Accordingly, patients with MS will sometimes view supplementation with PUFAs as a *reasonable gamble*, despite the lack of definitive evidence. It is easy to understand how the data are simultaneously compelling for some patients and unconvincing for many health professionals.

By weight, the richest sources of LA include sunflower oil, soybean oil, corn oil, walnut oil, wheat germ oil, grapeseed oil, and safflower oil. The richest sources of GLA include evening primrose oil, blackcurrant oil, borage seed oil, and spirulina. Rich sources of ALA include flaxseed oil, canola oil, and walnut oil. Some oils, such as walnut oil and flaxseed oil, contain relatively high levels of both LA and ALA. Rich sources of EPA and DHA include the fish oils found in salmon, Atlantic herring, Atlantic mackerel, bluefin tuna, sardine, and cod liver.[19] Additional information about many of these supplements can be found alphabetically in the main body of this guide.

The amount of EPA and DHA used in the large clinical trial described above[11] would be difficult to obtain from dietary sources. Indeed, it would require approximately one and a half servings of salmon or other fish per day. In addition to being impractical, such a diet may raise concerns regarding contaminants, such as mercury, especially among some populations, including pregnant women or women who might become pregnant.[20]

Unfortunately, the dietary supplement industry is insufficiently regulated, and the risk of contamination may also be significant with supplementation. Those looking to supplement their diet with PUFAs in the quantities that have been studied may want to seek high-quality sources that have been independently tested to assure purity.

References

1. Esparza ML, Sasaki S, Kesteloot H. Nutrition, latitude, and multiple sclerosis mortality: an ecologic study. *Am J Epidemiol* 1995;142(7):733–737.

2. Calder P. Dietary fatty acids and lymphocyte function. Proceedings of the Nutrition Society. 1998;57:487–502.

3. Gallai V, Sarchielli P, Trequattrini A, et al. Cytokine secretion and eicosanoid production in the peripheral blood mononuclear cells of MS patients undergoing dietary supplementation with n-3 polyunsaturated fatty acids. *J Neuroimmunol* 1995;56(2):143–153.

4. Harbige LS. Dietary n-6 and n-3 fatty acids in immunity and antoimmune disease. *Proc Nutr Soc* 1998;57(4):555–562.

5. Nordvik I, Myhr KM, Nyland H, Bjerve KS. Effect of dietary advice and n-3 supplementation in newly diagnosed MS patients. *Acta Neurol Scand* 2000;102(3):143–149.

6. Swank RL. Multiple sclerosis: fat-oil relationship. *Nutrition* 1991;7(5): 368–376.

7.   Fitzgerald G. Harbige LS, Forti A, Crawford MA. The effect of nutritional counseling on diet and plasma EFA status in multiple sclerosis patients over 3 years. *Hum Nutr Appl Nutr* 1987:41(5):297–310.

8.   Goldberg P, Fleming MC, Picard EH. Multiple sclerosis: decreased relapse rate through dietary supplementation with calcium, magnesium and vitamin D. *Med Hypotheses* 1986;21(2):193–200.

9.   Horrobin DF. Multiple sclerosis: the rational basis for treatment with colchicine and evening primrose oil. *Med Hypotheses* 1979;5(3):365–378.

10. Meyer-Rienecker JH, Jenssen HL, Kohler H, Field EJ, Shenton BK. Effect of gamma-linolenate in multiple sclerosis. *Lancet* 1976;2(7992):966.

11. Bates D, Cartlidge NE, Franch JM, et al. A double-blind controlled trial of long chain n-3 polyunsaturated fatty acids in the treatment of multiple sclerosis. *J Neurol Neurosurg Psychiatry* 1989;52(1):18–22.

12. Paty DW. Double-blind trial of linoleic acid in multiple sclerosis. *Arch Neurol* 1983;40(11):693–694.

13. Bates D, Fawcett PR, Shaw DA, Weightman D. Polyunsaturated fatty acids in treatment of acute remitting multiple sclerosis. *Br Med J* 1978;2:1390–1391.

14. Millar JH, Zilkha KJ, Langman MJ, et al. Double-blind trial of linoleate supplementation of the diet in multiple sclerosis. *Br Med J* 1973; 1(5856):765–768.

15. Weinstock-Guttman B, Baier M, Feichter J, et al. A randomized study of low fat diet with omega-3 fatty acid supplementation in patients with relapsing-remitting multiple sclerosis. *Neurology* 2003;60S:A151.

16. Wingerchuk DM, Noseworthy JH. Randomized controlled trials to assess therapies for multiple sclerosis. *Neurology* 2002;58(8 Suppl 4):S40–48.

17. Dworkin RH, Bates D, Millar JH, Paty DW. Linoleic acid and multiple sclerosis: a reanalysis of three double-blind trials. *Neurology* 1984; 34(11):1441–1445.

18. Bowling AC, Stewart TM. Current complementary and alternative therapies of multiple sclerosis. *Curr Treatment Options Neurol* 2003;5:55–68.

19. USDA National Nutrient Database for Standard Reference, Release 15 [program] 2003.

20. USFDA. FDA announces advisory on methyl mercury in fish. FDA Talk Paper [online]. Available at: http://www.fda.gov/bbs/topics/ANSWERS/2001/ANS01065.html. Accessed June 6, 2003.

Appendix 2—Vitamins and Minerals: Recommended Daily Allowances (RDAs), Adequate Intakes (AIs), and Tolerable Upper Intake Levels (ULs)

| | RDA/AI[1] | | | | |
	Men	Women	Pregnant	Lactating	UL[2]
Vitamins					
Biotin (Vitamin H)	30 mcg	30 mcg	30 mcg	35 mcg	ND[3]
Choline	550 mg	425 mg	450 mg	550 mg	3.5 g
Cobalamin (Vitamin B12)	2.4 mcg	2.4 mcg	2.6 mcg	2.8 mcg	ND[3]
Folate (Vitamin B9)	400 mcg	400 mcg	600 mcg	500 mcg	1000 mcg
Niacin (Vitamin B3)	16 mg	14 mg	18 mg	17 mg	35 mg
Pantothenic acid (Vitamin B5)	5 mg	5 mg	6 mg	7 mg	ND
Pyridoxine (Vitamin B6)	1.3 mg[4]	1.3 mg[5]	1.9 mg	2.9 mg	100 mg
Riboflavin (Vitamin B2)	1.3 mg	1.1 mg	1.4 mg	1.6 mg	ND
Thiamin (Vitamin B1)	1.2 mg	1.1 mg	1.4 mg	1.4 mg	ND

(continued on next page)

	RDA/AI[1]				UL[2]
	Men	Women	Pregnant	Lactating	
Vitamins (continued)					
Vitamin A	~3000 IU (900 mcg)	~2300 IU (700 mcg)	~2500 IU (770 mcg)	~4300 IU (1300 mcg)	~10,000 IU (3000 mcg)
Vitamin C	90 mg	75 mg	85 mg	120 mg	2000 mg
Vitamin D	200 IU (5 mcg[6])	200 IU (5 mcg[7])	200 IU (5 mcg)	200 IU (5 mcg)	2000 IU (50 mcg)
Vitamin E[8]	22 IU (15 mg)	22 IU (15 mg)	22 IU (15 mg)	28 IU (19 mg)	1500 IU (1000 mg)
Vitamin K	120 mcg	90 mcg	90 mcg	90 mcg	ND[3]
Minerals					
Calcium	1000 mg[9]	1000 mg[10]	1000 mg	1000 mg	2.5 g
Chromium	35 mcg[11]	25 mcg[12]	30 mcg	45 mcg	ND[3]
Copper	900 mcg	900 mcg	1000 mcg	1300 mcg	10,000 mcg
Fluoride	4 mg	3 mg	3 mg	3 mg	10 mg
Iodine	150 mcg	150 mcg	220 mcg	290 mcg	1100 mcg
Iron	8 mg	18 mg[13]	27 mg	9 mg	45 mg
Magnesium	420 mg[14]	310 mg[15]	350 mg[16]	310 mg[17]	350 mg
Manganese	2.3 mg	1.8 mg	2.0 mg	2.6 mg	11 mg
Molybdenum	45 mcg	45 mcg	50 mcg	50 mcg	2000 mcg
Phosphorus	700 mg	700 mg	700 mg	700 mg	4 g[18]
Selenium	55 mcg	55mcg	60 mcg	70 mcg	400 mcg
Zinc	11 mg	8 mg	11 mg	12 mg	40 mg

1. This table is taken from the DRI reports; see www.nap.edu. See also, http://www.nin.ca/public_html/En/pdf/dri.pdf. Recommended Daily Allowances (RDA) and Adequate Intakes (AI) may both be used as goals for individual intake. RDA refers to the needs of almost all (97–98%) individuals in a group. AI refers to the amount believed to cover the needs of all individuals in the group, but lack of data or uncertainty prevent stating with confidence the percentage of individuals covered. RDA appears in italics. Data provided refers to daily amounts and is for men and woman 19–70 years unless otherwise indicated.

2. UL refers to the Tolerable Upper Intake Level, which is the maximum level of daily nutrient intake that is likely to pose no risk of adverse effects.

3. ND indicates "not determinable" due to lack of data of adverse effects. This indicates concern with regard to lack of ability to handle excess amounts. Source of intake should be from food only to prevent high levels of intake.

4. Data provided are for men 19–50 years. For men 51 years and over, the AI is 1.7 mg.

5. Data provided are for women 19–50 years. For women 51 years and over, the AI is 1.5 mg.

6. Data provided are for men 19–50 years. For men 51–70, the AI is 10 mcg; for men 71 and over, the AI is 15 mcg.

7. Data provided are for women 19–50 years. For women 51–70, the AI is 10 mcg; for women 71 and over, the AI is 15 mcg.

8. Values shown are for alpha-tocopherol. For calculating RDAs, natural vitamin E (d-alpha-tocopherol) in IUs can be convered to alpha-tocopherol in mg by multiplying by 0.67; synthetic vitamin E (d,1–alpha-tocopherol or all-rac-alpha-tocopherol) in IU can be converted to alpha-tocopherol in mg by multiplying by 0.45. UL is 1100 IU for synthetic vitamin E and 1500 IU for natural vitamin E.

9. Data provided are for men 19–50 years. For men 51 and over, the AI is 1200 mg.

10. Data provided are for women 19–50 years. For women 51 and over, the AI is 1200 mg.

11. Data provided are for men 19–50 years. For men 51 and over, the AI is 30 mcg.

12. Data provided are for women 19–30 years. For women 51 years and over, the AI is 20 mcg.

13. Data provided are for women 19–50 years. For women 51 years and over, the RDA is 8 mg.

14. Data provided are for men 31 and over. For men 19–30 years, the RDA is 400 mg.

15. Data provided are for women 19 to 30 years old. For women 31 years and over, the RDA is 320 mg.

16. Data provided are for pregnant women 19 to 30 years old. For pregnant women 31 years and over, the RDA is 360 mg.

17. Data provided are for lactating women 19 to 30 years old. For lactating women 31 years and over, the RDA is 320 mg.

18. Data provided are for men and women 19 to 70 years old. For men and women 71 years or over, the UL is 3 g. For pregnant women, the UL is 3.5 g, and for lactating women, the UL is 4 g.

Index